THE Safe & Effective
eXercise PROGRAM

THE Safe & Effective eXercise PROGRAM

Don't Just Do it, Do it Better

Sam Banola

iUniverse, Inc.
New York Lincoln Shanghai

THE Safe & Effective eXercise PROGRAM
Don't Just Do it, Do it Better

iUniverse books may be ordered through booksellers or by contacting:

iUniverse
2021 Pine Lake Road, Suite 100
Lincoln, NE 68512
www.iuniverse.com
1-800-Authors (1-800-288-4677)

ISBN-13: 978-0-595-37659-9 (pbk)
ISBN-13: 978-0-595-82045-0 (ebk)
ISBN-10: 0-595-37659-2 (pbk)
ISBN-10: 0-595-82045-X (ebk)

Printed in the United States of America

The author does not claim that the information provided will prevent or cure any diseases, nor is he responsible for any injuries or illnesses that anyone may experience while taking part in any of the activities related to the program. It is not uncommon for old injuries to arise when one places a higher physical demand on their body. Therefore, it is recommended that anyone considering an exercise program consults with their physician (and/or fitness professional) about whether or not they may have any limitations or restrictions. There is always a risk of injury or even the possibility of death from partaking in an exercise program (although there is an even greater chance of preventing premature death and chronic lifestyle related diseases). The author also clearly states that he is not a registered dietician or nutritionist and therefore does not recommend any specific nutrient intake requirements. Rather he has provided you with some of the necessary information (education) to assist you in making better (healthier) choices in improving the quality of your food intake for the purpose of weight control. You should therefore consider all guideline and menu suggestions in this book to be just that, guidelines. You are to ultimately make the final decision as to what foods you put in your body (although many of you may benefit greatly by following the guidelines). If you have any extraordinary circumstances such as a metabolic disorder or cancer, it is recommended that you consult with a dietician as to what would be the best options for you.

Contents

Preface

This book is going to be your guide in taking ownership of your body and your life. You will learn exactly what you need to know to attain the results you are looking for. I want you to think of this as your personal owner's manual. Our parents never received one when we were born, and we were not given one when we first learned to read. Nearly everything we can purchase comes with some type of directions, yet when it comes to our body we are just expected to figure things out for ourselves. While the information has always been out there, judging from the average American's current state of health, the message has gotten lost.

This book is going to help you find your way. How many of you have personally experienced failure on one type of program or another? If you have not experienced this yourself, I can guarantee you at least know someone who has. There may have been some short term success, but in the end, the result is almost always the same.

It is time to put an end to this. It is time to stop aimlessly "trying" these short term programs that are impossible to follow for the rest of your life. You need to learn how to fuel your body properly and how to use it to its fullest potential. It is my belief that the information you are about to receive will allow you to break free from this ridiculous pattern and take control of your health.

Unless you have been a client of mine, you probably have not heard of me. I am not now, nor have I ever been a celebrity trainer. One does not need to be famous or train celebrities to have the status of a great trainer. There are many out there who you never have and probably never will hear of. This does not mean they are not successful in helping their clients attain results. They are doing the same job I have been doing for the past 9 years. This book is just a way for me to help more individuals than I could ever possibly reach in a one on one situation. My focus has always been on teaching ordinary everyday people what they need to know to get the results they desire. Over the years I have worked with these individuals to come up with strategies to implement changes into their lives. This book lists the 4 most important actions you must take to be successful with your efforts. If you use the strategies described in this book to create your exercise program, I am confident that you will be able to follow through with these 4 actions and reach your desired goal.

Most Americans are losing control, not just of our waistlines, but control of our lives. Many of us these days feel we have less and less time, and more to do in that time. Now, more than ever, we need to start taking better care of ourselves. Many parents worry about taking care of their family, so they devote themselves to their careers so they can provide for their family, financially. Others work to make as much as they can in hopes of one day being able to enjoy retirement. Unfortunately, if you don't take care of yourself now, you might not be around long enough to enjoy any of it.

Prioritizing and simplifying our lives can create more time for the important stuff. This is one of the first steps this book will take you through during the process of educating you on the truth about creating a lifelong weight maintenance program. Many of the diets that have come out in the past have failed the majority of the population.

Why have these plans failed us? Because many of the "diet gurus" have taken extreme positions in what they believe is best for us. Taking these positions, has allowed them to create a simple answer to our problems. We have followed them blindly because that "simple" answer seems so, well—simple. First, it was low fat, and now low carb is the way to go. What you need to know, and what you will learn in this book, is that the answer lies somewhere in between. Both the low fat and low carb camps have some truths to their arguments. However, we need to filter out much of what we have heard and focus on what has been scientifically proven to create a sound program. The fact is, not all fats are bad for you, some are absolutely essential. The same goes for carbohydrates; your body needs them to function properly. You just need to take in the right ones while eliminating the simple and processed ones.

If you live in the United States, the odds are that you are (at least to some degree) overweight. Americans need to wake up to this fact, and stop jumping on board with the latest fad diet program before they learn the facts. There have been more fads diets in the last 20 years than you could imagine. One thing you will learn in this book is what kind of results you should expect out of a well planned weight maintenance program. A well planned program should focus on creating a reduction in body fat more than just pure weight loss. Although this process does not occur as fast as the *48 HR miracle diet* ™ or the 30 pounds in 30 days flyers you sometimes see posted on a utility pole, the weight won't come back like it would with those plans either. Those types of plans do not create permanent weight loss. A well planned program should create a weight loss of 1–2 lbs per week or 50–100lbs in a year. This of course depends upon how closely you follow your program, but the results you get will last as long as you chose to have them last.

My responsibility as a fitness professional is to educate and empower my clients while helping them reach their goal. Part of this process is teaching them what actually works so they can eventually learn how to exercise properly and be successful on their own. This book has been created for the purpose of allowing you to benefit in the same way. This is not just information I have learned over the years, or read in a book or a journal. These are the very principles and techniques I have applied to myself as well as my clients. I have seen how great these techniques can work when followed correctly. I encourage you to learn these as well.

This book is meant to be a reference guide to steer you in the right direction towards a path of better health and fitness. I have not attempted to re-invent the wheel with this book, rather I have sifted through the research of some of the most knowledgeable people in the field and condensed this information into a simplified, what you need to know format, of what I believe is the most sensible approach to weight management, fat loss, and lifestyle adjustment.

Chapter 1

The Diet Industry

Chapter Highlights:
- Many of the "fad" diets are flawed and will lead you to failure.
- How diets can affect your metabolism and what you really lose.
- Our fast pace lifestyle has affected the quality of our lives.

How do you feel about yourself and your appearance? How do you feel at that moment just before you step into the shower, when you have taken off your clothes and you are standing there naked in front of the mirror? Would you like to change what you see? Do you believe that it is possible? Many people I have come across are on their last string of hope, they are willing to try just about anything or give up altogether. A lot of companies know this too. These companies know you want to change that person in the mirror. They also know if they make some (empty) promise, they can make millions. Some people are so desperate; they are willing to pay for the latest weight loss device or supplement, especially if it claims fast and easy results. Unfortunately, much of the information out there is, at best, easily misunderstood, and at worst it could possibly be harmful to your health. There are a lot of gimmicks out there, how much of your money have you donated to the multi-billion dollar a year weight loss industry?

Think about how many diets you have tried, how much weight have you lost? If your answer is, lost a few pounds, gained them back, you're not alone. If you added up all the pounds you've lost, it may be close to or in excess of your current body weight. Does this mean you are a failure at losing weight? Is this just the way you are supposed be? Probably not. Many of the Fad diets set you up for failure. They have a common theme—<u>calorie deprivation</u>. It does not matter whether it is the *Cabbage Soup diet*™, *Scarsdale diet*™, *Grapefruit diet*™, *Hollywood 48hr Miracle Diet*™, or maybe even the pop-up add I received on my computer while writing this book. It claimed I could lose weight while sitting at my computer and I would not have to alter my diet or exercise. Many of these diets whether there is a "magic" herbal pill involved or not, are some form of a calorie deprivation plan. They will give you a quick initial weight loss only to be followed by a quick weight gain. Notice I did not say fat loss, which is really the key to being successful. Much of the weight lost on these plans comes from water and muscle. When you restrict calories, your body actually believes it is being starved. The metabolism slows down to prepare the body for lower calorie intake. When your metabolism slows down three important things happen to you.

(1. It makes it harder for you to lose weight. A slower metabolism means fewer calories burned while you are exercising, working, sleeping, or anything else.

(2. It makes it easier to store fat; this is how your body would get you through a real food crisis.

(3. Once you go off the plan, you will more than likely gain your weight back and then some. This occurs because you return to your old eating habits with a new, slower metabolism.

This is scientifically proven information. **The National Institute of Health** conducted a study and their research found that 90% of those who lose weight on a medically supervised diet will regain that weight within three years. I have personally seen some do that sooner and gain more than what they originally lost, so don't think something like *MediFast*™ might be your solution. Diet alone is not the solution for the current obesity epidemic.

Take your local national chain weight loss center for example. Jennifer and her husband Craig are concerned about the weight they have put on in the past year. They feel it is necessary for them to have their weight watched. Let's follow Jennifer's experience to see what happens. When Jenny comes in to have a plan set up, she is given a specific number of calories or points for her daily intake. She is allowed to eat whatever she wants as long as she stays in the prescribed range. The consultant who prescribes this plan tells Jenny this will allow for more flexibility in her daily food choices. I have worked with clients who were on these plans. Many of them were very excited to hear that they can eat just about anything, until they learned the facts. Eating a low calorie intake consisting of highly processed foods and simple carbohydrates may help them lose some weight at first, but will do nothing for improving their health because the foods they are eating are basically empty calories. On several occasions I have asked these clients to record their food intake so I could see what foods they were eating. Many times they were way out of balance in terms of macronutrients (proteins, carbohydrates, and fats). I'm not saying you have to be perfect, but if you want to lose weight and improve your health you must choose quality foods such as lean proteins, whole grains, fruits, and vegetables that provide vitamins and minerals in their natural form.

Regardless, let's say our Jenny is on the plan, and after two weeks she is down 9 lbs. Some nice initial progress from the large calorie deficit they created. After four weeks she is only down 2 more lbs, so they readjust her plan with fewer points or calories. The following week Jenny is down another 6 lbs. Although she is happy with 17 lbs in five weeks, she feels hungry, deprived, and irritable, but is determined to do this right. After two more weeks and no more weight loss she is now getting discouraged and really hungry. Feeling more tempted to have something "special" to reward herself for her achievement of losing 17 lbs, Jenny decides to go out and eat (pizza, ice cream…). She felt she worked hard to get there and she knows she can't keep eating like this forever; maybe having her favorite comfort food every now and then will work out. Unfortunately, after that first little splurge, it becomes harder to stay with the plan. She convinces herself she is happy with what she achieved and that she can return to some of her old "normal" eating habits. After a few weeks of "normal" eating with a slower metabolism Jenny has gained 5 lbs back. After a few months she has added another 8 lbs and is almost at her initial starting weight.

Is this the typical pattern for you? Maybe it's time to stop blaming yourself for the failures and realize many of the plans are flawed. The most important thing to note from the above paragraph is that "She can't keep eating like this forever". If you want a plan to work, you better find one that you can do for the rest of your life; it should become a part of your life.

You might wonder why or how does your metabolism slow down when you restrict calories. One reason is, when you do not take in enough calories to maintain basic functions, your body begins to break down tissues to get what it needs. If you are on a very "low carb" diet, it is difficult to get in enough calories. This creates a state of "food crisis" in which your body is being stressed. This stress causes an increase in the hormone cortisol. There are two negative effects of this hormone. First, this stress hormone will promote fat storage. This fat usually gets stored in the abdominal region as intramuscular fat. This is a bit different than subcutaneous (under the skin) fat and has more health risks associated with it. Second, cortisol sets off a catabolic process. Catabolism is the process of breaking down tissues. By breaking down muscle tissue and sending amino acids into the blood stream, the body can convert these amino acids into the much needed glucose. (Glucose is what all food is broken down into so the body can use it as fuel.) Since your body is not taking enough fuel in the form of carbohydrates, it has found another way to make this preferred energy source.

Just to recap and fully explain the above process before we move on. When you ingest carbohydrates, your body breaks them down into glucose. Glucose is basically sugar in your blood which is either used for energy or stored. At first, unused glucose gets stored into the muscle tissue and liver in the form of glycogen. (Glycogen is the stored form of glucose.) Excess glucose in your system is not something you want if you are trying to lose fat. If you take in more than you need it can reduce your body's ability to burn fat and it can also be converted into and stored as fat. Carbohydrates in the form of muscle glycogen stores are the most readily broken down for energy. This is what gets you through your day and all your activities. When someone first goes on a low carb diet, their body uses it's stored glycogen for energy. This will not last too long. When these supplies get low it is common for dieters to feel lethargic and irritable. Next the body goes into the catabolic process already described. By breaking down muscle glycogen as well as muscle proteins for energy, much of the weight lost on a low carb plan, which is really a low calorie plan in disguise, is not from fat. In fact along with each gram of glycogen removed from muscle goes 2.4 grams of water (up to 70% of weight loss).The following is an excerpt from an excellent article written by Phil Kaplan entitled, "The Low-Carb Lunacy".

When you consume a healthful diet complete with proteins, carbs and fats, carbohydrates are broken down into glucose. Some of that glucose is transported and stored in the muscle as "glycogen" and used to produce energy that fuels muscle contraction. An understanding of that simple fact, that carbohydrates are the source of muscle fuel, should raise an immediate red flag toward anything that suggests nearly eliminating carbs.

Some of the carbs you eat ultimately wind up stored as liver glycogen. The liver acts as sort of a "pump" for blood sugar. The brain burns more calories than any other organ in your body and uses glucose as its primary source of fuel. As brain activity results in "burning" of blood glucose, the liver accesses its glycogen stores to keep blood glucose in adequate supply. Again, as you expend glycogen, the carbs you ingest replenish your supply.

Cut Carbs? At First You'll Do Fine, But…
At first, when you cut way back on carbs, you're doing just fine. You have glycogen stored. After a day or two, you're depleting your stored glycogen and you're not replacing it. Your body shortly thereafter begins producing ketone bodies.

Ketones are intermediaries in the process of metabolizing fat that are found in abnormal amounts in the blood and urine during periods of metabolic impairment. Give up all of your stored glycogen without replacing it and you're likely going to be in such a state. Atkins leads you to believe that the presence of these ketone bodies indicates ongoing fat release. He also assures you that they feed the brain. That is partially true. Here are just a few of the issues that he neglects to address:

1. Extended periods of ketosis affect the chemical composition of the blood in such a way that you increase risk of cardiac incident (blood ketoacidosis).

2. In a state of ketoacidosis, carbon dioxide accumulates in the tissues. Oxygen delivery to the cells is impaired. This can lead to a wide range of disastrous consequences ranging from respiratory ailments to metabolic illness.

3. Toxic ammonia buildup resulting from severe cases of ketoacidosis can be lethal.

I believe all the low-carb gurus neglect to share this information with their readers. They also neglect to tell you the liver is called into play to "filter" the abnormal chemicals building up in the blood, leading to a residual buildup of uric acid. Interestingly enough, this uric acid accumulation can lead to the formation of kidney stones.

But Don't You Lose Weight?
In confronting Atkins, I asked if he agrees that calorie deprivation leads to metabolic slowdown. "Absolutely." I then expressed my concern that his book encourages people to judge their progress by pounds. "If muscle is lost, metabolism slows, yet the scale would indicate weight reduction. Isn't this the major problem with the conventional calorie deprivation diets?" I followed with, "Isn't it true that the initial weight lost on your diet will be primarily water loss, temporary and meaningless in hope of long-term weight reduction?"

Atkins started to deny it. I continued, "I'm not a doctor, so I hope you'll correct me if I'm wrong. I was led to believe that one gram of glycogen attracts 2.4 grams of water, thus if you hold less glycogen in muscle due to carb restriction, it's a given there will be

> *substantial water loss." Again I asked, "So isn't the initial weight loss primarily water loss?" He started to grow irritated, but I heard the words come out, "Well, yeah, maybe the initial weight loss."*

The article ends by explaining that by going into a carb-restrictive plan you, by default end up in a calorie deprived state. Ironically, this happens to be the reason that Dr. Atkins sites as to why other diets have failed America. This article can be found in (Personal Fitness Professional July, 2000 p32–35) Phil Kaplan also follows up the article in 2002 after Dr. Atkins death to point out the fact that he actually applauds Dr. Atkins for challenging the medical establishment and making us question what is really making us fat.

As I have already explained, muscle glycogen and proteins are lost on a calorie restrictive diet. When this occurs muscle mass gets reduced and the metabolism will slow. You may be wondering, what do I care as long as I lose weight. What is this metabolism thing you keep mentioning anyway? Think of your metabolism as your body's engine. When you give it high quality fuel (food) at regular intervals you can keep it running on all cylinders. This engine is responsible for burning around 75% of your daily calorie output. When you eat calories, they are converted into fuel to perform your daily tasks. If you take away a cylinder or two by losing muscle mass, you will reduce your daily calorie output. On the other hand you can also increase the size of this engine. Muscle is an active tissue and for each pound of muscle gained, it can change the metabolic rate by anywhere from 35–100 calories depending on the individual. Just for reference 100 calories per day x 365 days equates to 36500 calories in a year. If we divide this 36500 calories by/3500 calories per lb = we get 10.42 lbs.

Obviously, you can see from the above example, as few as 100 calories per day can work for you or against you in a big way. Unfortunately, for many Americans it has gone against them over the last 20 years. Slight changes to our lifestyle, such as remote controls for the TV and Stereo, video game systems and many other convenience devices have allowed us to become less active. Think of your lifespan, when you were younger, maybe some of these conveniences were around, maybe not. I guarantee at least one thing has changed for most of us, our activity levels. As we get older we tend to become less active. When you were in grade school and high school you may not have played a sport but at least you had recess and gym class to get you up and moving during the day. This is more than we can say for our kids now, which is going to create one of the unhealthiest generations ever. Did you know that the rate of obesity in children has skyrocketed in the past 25 years? The number of children considered severely obese has doubled from 1 in 14 to 1 in 7. I guess we could find someone to blame for this, let's blame video games. That's what we do these days right, who wants to take responsibility for their actions anymore.

We have all heard the case of the guy who discovered he was fat, and realized McDonalds never told him not to eat there 3 times a day. They made him fat; therefore they owe him a lot of money. Maybe it's time we start to take ownership of our problems. Maybe we need to admit that we as a society have shown kids that exercise is not that important. The **Centers For Disease Control** estimates the number of schools that offer daily physical education has dropped by over one third during the past 10 years. Our priorities are way off base. When it comes to budgets physical education is usually one of the first programs cut. Meanwhile administrators have allowed corporations to invade our schools with machines dispensing drinks with 11 spoons of sugar per can. The latest reports show that when kids drink more than one soda per day it increases the risk of obesity, diabetes, caffeine dependency, cavities, and weakened bones. How many articles about obesity and children do we have to see before serious action is taken?

The **American Academy of Pediatrics** believes kids now need body-mass checkups to help identify and prevent obesity. They are concerned about the prevalence of obesity and obesity-related disorders in children. They also believe that obesity-related health costs may be greater than that of smoking.

As some of you have grown older maybe you have kept up with some recreational activities despite the fact you started your first job (sitting at a desk) and more time was dedicated to work, and less for play/activity. But, once you had kids, your free time was reduced even further. This pattern of decreasing activity needs to be changed, and if you do not break the cycle in some way, you will feel and look much older than you should. Our kids follow our example; they are starting this pattern at a younger age due in part to the school systems. How and when do you think they will ever change this pattern if you as a parent do not exercise, eat right and value your health?

If you would really like to break the cycle and change that person you see in the mirror, you need to get started with a sound program. The proper way to burn fat and lose weight is to eat a balanced diet with adequate calorie intake to prevent the slowing of the metabolism. If you create a moderate gap between calories in and calories out you can safely create a fat loss of 1–2 pounds per week

(50–100 in a year is pretty good). That is about as fast as the body can metabolize fat, anything more will probably be water or muscle tissue lost. That is why people gain the weight back when they go on one of those plans that claim to give you rapid weight loss. It's not so much about achieving a certain weight as it is about reducing body fat, and eating for optimal nutrition and metabolic balance.

Chapter 2

Change
What are the ingredients to success and what holds us back?

Chapter Highlights:

- Setting realistic and clearly defined goals is essential to your success.
- Hold yourself accountable for your actions or find someone who will.
- Values and beliefs will control your actions, make sure you know what yours are.

"In order to change one must hurt so much you have to, learn so much you want to, receive so much you're able to." *Unknown (to me)* This book is about change. Change in the way you think, eat, exercise, basically a change in the way you live. If you bought this book it may well be because you "hurt so much" and you know you need to make a change. Now that you have taken that first crucial step, it is time to learn what you need to know so you are able to make this change successfully.

What will make your change process a successful one? **Attitude**. More of this battle is in your head than you realize. As a trainer I have to put a lot of trust in my client's ability to follow the plan I design for them. Even with the perfect cardiovascular, resistance training, and nutrition plan, results will be limited if it is not followed consistently. Even if I see them 3 times per week, I am not there to see what they are doing during the other 165 hours of that 7-day period. I can only ensure the quality of the workouts I am there to administer. This is why establishing the proper attitude in my clients is one of the keys to their success. Part of my business depends upon them getting results and others noticing and asking how they did it. So I better believe in what I teach and live by the guidelines I have developed. Only then can my clients have faith in the information I give them. Establishing this faith and getting a client into the proper mindset is the first step in undertaking a lifestyle adjustment program. This is done before they take their first step onto any treadmill. We work on establishing realistic goals and recognition of why they want to achieve a particular goal. This is an important step for you to do for yourself as well.

Answer these questions:

What is your main long-term goal? Is your health your main concern, or is your appearance more of an issue. (In 6 months–1 year where would you like to be?)

_____

   Now break it down into 2 or more short-term goals:
   (In 1–3 months, what initial changes would you like to see?)
   These goals should be specific and measurable i.e. lose a specific clothing size, increase in strength or flexibility, get a compliment.

   _____

   _____

Why do you want to achieve your particular goals?_____

_____

What will achieving your goals do for you, and why are they important? (Think about what new things you will be able to do when you achieve your goal)_____

_____

How will you feel when you reach these goals?_____

_____

Is this all worth it? (Is the effort worth the payoff?)_____

_____

Before you answer, remember that there are always tradeoffs. You will have to make some sacrifices. Make a list of all the pros and cons:

_____   _____   _____   _____

_____   _____   _____   _____

The pros may not always outweigh the cons. You may have reasons not to adopt a lifestyle adjustment program. Some may be obvious and some may not. Maybe creating a change will disrupt family life, or how those around you feel. The new you may make them uncomfortable in some way. On that note, don't worry about the insecure people who try to get you to "live a little". They try to sabotage you because they do not feel comfortable about themselves. You will need to really think this through—be completely honest with yourself because you have no one else to fool. If you are okay will the possible outcomes, this means that the pros do outweigh the cons and your lifestyle adjustment program should be "worth it."

The next question is:

Are you willing to do whatever it takes to achieve your goals?

Think about the circumstances that may have held you back in the past and how you can better plan to overcome these obstacles. You may want to make a list of the things that prevented you from being successful in the past. A better list would contain your current barriers to success and behavioral strategies you can apply to overcome them.

1. If you have a busy schedule and do not have time to cook dinner more than 3 nights per week. Behavior Plan—Cook excess portions of meals on those nights put them in containers and freeze them so you can have a good, quick and easy meal on the other nights.

2. Something always comes up during the day and takes away from the time you planned on exercising. Behavioral Plan—Set the alarm earlier and do your workout first thing in the morning.

Other behavioral plans include: recording your workouts and planning to hit a certain number each week or month, journaling your food intake and setting a goal of 4–6 meals per day, and weighing out your food portions if you are not sure of what they should be.

List any other obstacles that apply to you here:

_____

_____

Once you identify them, you can create a plan of attack.

Do you have someone to share these goals with or to support you in your journey? This can be very helpful in achieving your goals. Support could come from a spouse, family member, or friend—someone who can cheer you on or even participates in your lifestyle adjustment program. Support could even come from a personal trainer—someone who can give you proper guidance and hold you accountable.

It is important that you answer all of these questions before we move on. This information will be used to customize your program and remind you of why you are taking on this task.

Change does not need to be difficult—many perceive it to be much more difficult than it actually is. Part of the problem is that many people wait until their current situation becomes too painful or uncomfortable to maintain. Only then do they decide to do something about it. Motivation through pain, as great as it is, will only get you so far. As soon as the pain is gone the motivation may also disappear. That is why you should take the time to complete the previous questions. Once you see the benefits of your actions and what they will do for you in the future, 1, 5, or even 10 years from now, you should become excited about the possibilities. If that is not enough motivation for you, maybe you should think about what your future will be like 1, 5, or 10 years from now if you do not take any action to better your health. Do you really want to look and feel older than you should? When you take this point of view, you may decide it is well worth the effort it takes to create change.

Another key factor in getting results is **accountability**. The more frequently I see a client, the more opportunities I have to influence their decisions. They know that when they see me, they will have to report on their progress. That simple fact tends to lead to better results. To give yourself this same advantage, I suggest you find a way to hold yourself accountable or find someone as an accountability partner. You could hire a trainer, begin the program with a friend, or just keep a journal of your progress. One of my roles in working with a client is to help hold them accountable—I want to help them understand what they want to accomplish and to also know why they want that particular result. It is important that they fully understand what achieving that result can do for them and it is also important for me to know. If a client tells me she wants to lose 4 dress sizes, I want to know why. Just wanting to lose a few sizes is not always an important enough reason to do what it takes to reach that goal. If she wants to lose 4 dress sizes because she would like to surprise her husband and renew her wedding vows after 25 years, while wearing the same dress—that's a much more powerful reason. I can use this information to remind (motivate) her the first time she tells me she can't get up in the morning to do her cardio program.

What holds us back?

I'm sure we all know someone who does nothing but complain about their (*Fill in the blank*) (spouse, job, kids, car, weight, hair, etc.). If you have ever confronted them on their complaint, you're sure to have found that many of them are not planning on doing anything about it. The reason they do not take action is **fear**. They are not yet uncomfortable enough to do anything, and the fear of confronting a co-worker, leaving a job, arguing with their spouse, being in a new situation, is just too much. They have doubts about whether taking action will worsen their situation or better it. Eventually the time comes when they see taking action is worth the risk, or they come to better understand their situation. The following example is from an excellent article on motivation from Phil Kaplan:

> *"Let me share my experience in motivating an actual client. Meet Wayne. He took classes, sometimes 60-minute, sometimes 90-minute classes every day. Wayne hated mirrors. He didn't want to see his body. It was fat. It took courage for Wayne to dance around in a room where most participants were women and most were in better-than-average physical condition. What motivated him? Pain and fear, the greatest motivators in existence. I'm going to suggest you use those motivators and stimulate your clients' fears and emotional pains, at least momentarily. Before you condemn me for suggesting this, understand the power and virtue of my suggestion. Let me tell you about Wayne's progression to illustrate the outcome of a 'getting into the mind' motivational approach and then lead up to the concept of using pain as a motivator.*

> *"Wayne would gain and lose the same eight pounds. He tried diet after diet. Some days he'd feel the diet was working, others he was sure it wasn't. When he no longer sensed potential, he'd give up. Since he was already doing advanced aerobics classes and was overweight, he dreaded the thought of what would happen if he backed off on the aerobics. Why didn't he feel motivated to stick to the diet? He didn't feel any sense of potential. Why did he feel motivated to keep up his exercise? Fear! The fear of getting fatter was more painful than the thought of dancing around in front of 35 fit women, thus, he showed up for classes nearly everyday."* (How Do You Motivate Clients? **PFP** August 1999, pp. 18–19)

As you can see, pain and fear can be great motivators, but they can also hold us back. If you really want to create a change, you cannot be afraid of change. As I mentioned earlier, there are some tradeoffs, and you will have to make some sacrifices. This does not mean you will be worse off—you may really enjoy the benefits.

Have you ever heard the poem about the girl walking down the street who falls into a deep, deep sewer hole? You see, each day while walking home she turns down the same street and each day the cover is not on the hole. She does not see the hole and she falls in. It takes her hours to find her way out. After several occasions of falling in she gets better at finding her way out and it takes less and less time. Yet she still wastes time every day finding her way out of the hole. Finally, one day she decides to map out a new route and take a different street. This new street is a bit longer because it winds around the other one, but her walk home becomes much more enjoyable.

Life is about choosing your own path—the best one is not always the shortest, quickest, or easiest. Have you ever watched a horror movie and felt like reaching into the television and telling the character they are about to make a bad decision. You can't believe what they are about to do, but they do it anyway. These characters can be very predictable. Think about the first time you saw one of the sequels to the movie *Friday the 13th*™. During the scene when the character was getting chased through the woods by Jason, did you predict that they would trip and fall? Although you probably didn't write the script, you just knew, based on past performance, that these plots are very similar. Guess what? In many ways, so are the plots in your life. We do tend to be creatures of habit. It's just a matter of creating some good ones and dropping the bad ones. If you think about it, most people perform the same actions day in and day out. It is these actions that have led you to your current situation.

The way things happen in your life is not any less predictable than the way things happen to characters in horror movies. The problem is that many times you are so busy getting through it, you can't see what's coming next. Not being able to see what is coming next is the reason why many people make poor choices and fall into the same kinds of traps all the time. What you need to do is step back and look at your life from an outsider's point of view. Really take some time to analyze what you do, when you do it, and why you do the things you do. This new perspective will allow you to make better decisions so you can choose the right path for you—Instead of the one you had to take because you were not prepared.

So far we have learned that change is not that difficult, but getting over the fear of taking the first step can be. We have also learned that having the right mindset, the right "attitude" going into this process; will help you stay consistent with your plan. What we now need to understand is what controls your mindset? Why do you, and why would you, decide to take any particular action? Remember, you always have a choice in everything you do. According to Robert White in his book *Living an Extraordinary Life,* you make the choice that serves you best at the time. Meaning, based on current information, you choose to do X. You may later find out that you should have done Z, but you did not know that at the time. So again: Why do you make these choices? It all comes down to values and beliefs. You see, everyone has certain values and beliefs about everything. These are what cause us to take the actions that we take and what lead to the outcomes that are our lives. Sometimes it is these values and beliefs that keep you from achieving success.

Beliefs are things you accept as true. When you were younger you may have believed in Santa Claus or the Tooth Fairy. You were not born with this belief, someone made you believe it, and you later found out that the belief was false. I guarantee that some of you are still holding on to false beliefs. While these beliefs may be important to you for various reasons, some of them may be doing you harm. The following is a quote from Ayn Rand that I use at the beginning of my programs to emphasize this very point:

> *"As a human being, you have no choice about the fact you need a philosophy. Your only choice whether you define your philosophy by a conscious, rational, disciplined process of thought and scrupulously logical deliberation—or let your subconscious accumulate a junk heap of unwarranted conclusions, false generalizations, undefined contradictions, undigested slogans, unidentified wishes, doubts and fears, thrown together by change, but integrated by your subconscious into a kind of mongrel philosophy and fused into a single, solid weight: self-doubt, like a ball and chain in the place where your mind's wings have grown."*

Many of these false beliefs you may be holding on to were formed at a very young age, when you were highly susceptible to the influence of those around you. What if those people were not the most positive-thinking folks? Their negative attitudes most likely rubbed off on you in some way. If they defined you without fully knowing what you might be capable of, you may now be selling yourself short. Those beliefs are probably holding you back "like a ball and chain." What you need to do is analyze your belief system and see if this is the case. Just because you learned something a long time ago does not mean it is true. Did you know we once thought the world was flat? Did you know that doctors once believed bed rest was the best thing for a heart attack patient? It is now known that getting up and moving around is the best thing to do as soon as it can be done safely. Be open minded to things that may be different than what you are used to. If you are someone who has always had negative beliefs about yourself and your ability to change, or you have never felt yourself worthy of something positive, it is time to change that. Positive thinking will lead to positive actions, and it is these actions which will lead to your desired outcome.

Values are things you feel are important. Family, health, friends, money, and so forth, are all things that people value. Not everyone prioritizes them the same way, but we all set aside time and energy for these things we value. While the topic of values seems fairly straightforward, the tricky part is to look at your life and identify what your values actually are. Before you go on, write them down and prioritize them below:

1_____   3_____   5_____   7_____

2_____   4_____   6_____   8_____

Now you need to look a bit deeper. Remember, our values and beliefs determine our actions. Assign a percentage to the amount of time you spend on each of your values over the course of an average week. Do your percentages of time spent, or "actions," in regard to your values match up with the priority numbers you assigned above, or are you spending more of your time on values of lower priority?

If your actions and values do not match up properly, this will cause stress in your life. For example, if you wrote down "family" as your number one priority, but you work 60–70 hours a week and miss all of your kids' little league games that will cause some family problems. Maybe you are single and you value leisure time, but you also work long hours. You may not have the time to do the recreational activities you so much used to enjoy. You need to look at your list again. Do you really want to get back into mountain biking or would you rather have a higher income? If you really miss your biking, make some sacrifices so you can create the time to do it. Otherwise, quit making yourself feel bad about it and just admit you value money over leisure. It's okay, they are your values.

Now that you have some understanding of how values and beliefs will control your decision making process, you should use this information to take the appropriate actions. Decide what your goals are, what outcome you are looking for, and map out your plan. Just like the girl in the poem, you can choose to take a new path and stop falling into that hole.

Chapter 3

The Program
Putting your plan together

Chapter Highlights:

- Keeping your mind in the program.
- Deprogramming the message of the weight loss industry.
- The 4 steps to following this plan.

Before we get into the details of this program, there are a few things for you to keep in mind. Consistency and persistence are your two biggest allies in the quest for better health and fitness. You do not need to be perfect 100% of the time to achieve results. I have yet to see one person do their program perfectly. However, the ones who do well, when they do have a slip up, will always start over with their very next meal or workout. The all or nothing attitude will not serve you well. If you temporarily get off track, use it as a learning experience so you can do better the next time you are in that situation. Learning from mistakes and how to plan ahead for situations will be a major key to your success. If you are going to a party, barbecue, or some other event, you can almost always plan ahead and (for the most part) follow your program. For example, if you are going to an event scheduled for 3pm and you know there will not be many good choices of food to eat when you get there, you can get 3–4 quality meals in before 3pm. If you do this and then have one meal that day which was not ideal, this is really not that big of an issue. If you're eating 5 meals a day × 7 days a week, 1 or 2 not-so-great meals out of 35 is a small fraction. With your new "revved up" metabolism this will not stop your progress and you will not gain any significant weight. The only way this could become a problem is if these events happen all the time and you fail to plan for them or your other meals.

A tip for when you are in these situations: It is common for the smell of a food or sight of something to bring back memories of a pleasure it brought you at one time. That does not mean it will do this again. Many times people who react to these feelings realize they really did not really want "it". When they got "it", it really was nothing like "it" used to be. They did not even enjoy "it". Then they felt guilty about "it". If you think (about what "it" will do for you) before you act, you will be less likely to do "it", and if you decide take action, you should not feel guilty about "it".

Another important issue is the scale; do not let it control your mindset. It is perfectly normal to fluctuate a few pounds each day whether you follow your program perfectly or not—this is water weight. If you are a woman and are menstruating, you will be especially susceptible to this. What is important is that your weight trends downward over the course of time. This is a program you can stick with for life, so you do not need to worry about gaining it all back, ever. In fact, if you follow this program correctly, you will be able to eat more when you finish then when you started without packing on any pounds.

One last thing which applies to all aspects of your plan is this. It's going to take some work to get to where you want to be, but once you get there it takes less effort to sustain that level. Think about if you were trying to swim upstream; it requires more effort to get from point A to point B than it does to remain at point B once you arrive. Yes, you must still work to remain there, but only the dead fish float downstream.

Now that we have that out of the way, let's get into creating your plan for success. I'm sure most of you have read or been told that you should exercise and eat right for your health, appearance…We all know what we should do. We also know that burgers, fries, soda, and ice cream are all bad for us. So why don't we do what is best for us. As I mentioned in the previous chapter, it has a lot to do with our mindset. If we can change our thinking, we can change our bodies. Unfortunately, most of the diet industry does not want us to accomplish this. They know what you want to hear. "Lose weight without changing anything", "lose weight fast", "you don't need to change your eating if you take this magic pill", or "use our special exercise device and it will melt off the pounds". When most folks here those types of messages, they get hooked. Despite being skeptical, they want to believe in something. The industry has a special way of reeling in their catch too. The word "guaranteed" or "money back guarantee" is almost always in bold print. The usually low price along with the guarantee helps the buyer feel more at ease. The buyer thinks "what have I got to lose" and the industry has another catch. They know as long as they say it's guaranteed you will buy it and only a small percentage of you will return the product. What the buyer does not know is that most of these ads have very small print which states "results not typical".

We need to stop letting them program us by telling us what we want to hear, and we need to start listening to what we need hear. Hear are the cold hard facts: Most of you do need to change your food intake to improve your health. Most of you also need to exercise more than you currently do, or at least smarter than you currently do. There are no magic pills. Nearly all supplements are a complete waste of money (see appendix VII). The exercise devices you see on TV are sold on TV for a reason (so you cannot try it first). It is nearly impossible to find a really good piece of exercise equipment for less than $500 and many are over $1000, however, this would be money well spent. Think of it as an investment in yourself. And last but not least, if you put forth the effort towards a sound exercise program "results are typical"

It's unfortunate that the truth is not always enough to get someone excited enough about starting a program. This is what allows the frauds to exist. Realizing this, I'm going to use some of the advertising skills they would typically use. First, we need a hook. We need to create a plan with a catchy little zing. Something that will get your attention. What if we call this plan "The Great SEX Diet"? Now, we need to set some guidelines, some simple rules to follow for this plan. You know, just like the "industry" would say, "all you need to do is_____" and you will get incredible results. Well I have come up with four essential rules that must be followed to produce great results.

Rule # 1 **Eat nutritionally balanced meals every 3hrs to fuel your body and boost your metabolism.**
Rule # 2 **Perform your cardio workouts when glycogen stores are lower.**
Rule # 3 **Perform a periodized weight training program.**
Rule # 4 **You need to make sure you have SEX every night (minimum 5 per week) 2 hours before bedtime on an empty stomach.**

To make this program work optimally you must follow all of the rules. If you do not follow all of them you will not be doing the complete program (get the entire effect) and will limit your results. We will get into the specifics of rules 1–3 in the next few chapters. For now we are going to concentrate on rule # 4.

How's that for a plan? Think of how great this can be. You get improve your sex life, your health, and lose weight all at the same time. What a way to get your spouse involved with your program. You can tell them you need to do this to improve your health. If you do not have a significant other, it's okay. You can be just as successful on this program going solo. The key is that you follow those simple instructions along with the nutritional and exercise guidelines you will learn about in the following chapters.

SEX can be defined as two things. For those of you who got excited at the idea of this plan, I want you do go through with it. You will soon learn how this can improve more than just your figure. For those of you who do not approve of such an idea, that's okay too. SEX is an acronym for Safe and Effective eXercise. The safe and effective exercise you can and should do at night includes yoga, stretching, or just meditation. This can help you to improve flexibility, relax, and clear your mind before you go to bed. You may end up sleeping better and waking up with more energy.

> *Note: you probably would do best to avoid any strenuous exercise too close to bedtime, as it may disrupt your ability to sleep.*

Whichever interpretation you choose the reason for recommending that any-thing be done 2 hours before bed is that this is what some of the "magic pill" companies recommend. If you must do or take something 2 hours before bed on an empty stomach, this means you are not snacking after dinner. For example, if you go to bed at 10 p.m. and "do it" at 8 p.m., this means you should not have had anything to eat since 6 p.m. Snacking is one of the reasons so many people start to pack on the pounds. Nighttime snacking is usually the result of some other issue. It might be due to boredom, loneliness, or just some need to fill a void. The food will not do this, but it is a distraction. When someone follows the directions on the box of some "magic pill," it is not so much the pill working as it is the effect of not snacking at night. When following my plan you will have something else to fill this time at the end of the day. Combine this with eating balanced meals throughout the day and you will not feel nearly as hungry at this time either.

Option 1—There are many benefits to following this plan and actually having sex. Why should we have sex this frequently? In case you did not realize, sex is exercise. It is an activity that burns calories (60–155 per hour) and elevates the heart rate for a variable period of time, depending on the person. I'm not trying to get everyone to trade in their running shoes and hop into bed. However, if you were to have sex 3 times per week for a year, it would be the equivalent of running 75 miles (Susie Michelle Cortright, Jorbins.com, *The Health Benefits of Sex.*) That's a fair amount of exercise and calorie burning. For some, that may be more annual exercise than you currently do and would be a great start to improving your health. Although it's not quite enough to be your only form of exercise, it is a great way to burn some extra calories.

Burning calories is just one of many benefits of having sex on a regular and frequent basis. Sex can help you live longer, look younger, feel better, and get stronger. These are all proven facts from dozens of studies on couples in intimate relationships. As we all know, and as some of the studies point out, promiscuous sex can actually have the opposite effect, for several reasons. Nevertheless, studies have shown that sex can actually slow the aging process. Researchers found that men who had 2 orgasms per week lived 1.6 years longer than those who only had 1 per week. They also found that those who had 3 orgasms per week appeared 10 years younger than those who had only 1 or 2 per week *(Royal Edinburgh Hospital in Scotland, Dr. David Weeks)*. Others studies have shown that during sex the brain releases endorphins (feel-good chemicals), which ease pain. These are the same chemicals that give you the "runner's high" during regular exercise. There is even evidence that sex can improve the immune system. Couples who have sex 1–2 times per week increase the chemical compound immunoglobulin A, which protects the body against infections *(Wilkes University in Wilkes-Barre, Pa)*. Researchers have also found that sex increases the flow of testosterone, which strengthens bones and muscles. This is the very same hormone that athletes and bodybuilders sometimes inject to perform better. Maybe that's why Wilt Chamberlain was able to score so many points.

With all these benefits, it's a wonder we don't already partake more often. Unfortunately, many of us sometimes have the same reasons for not "doing it" as we do for not exercising. The good news is, sex can help exercise and exercise can help sex. That is one of the reasons I developed this plan. As you will learn in chapter 6, exercise can impact your life in many ways. First there are the obvious health benefits, then there are the ways it can help to structure and organize your life, but there is more. Increased muscle mass, decreased body fat, and feeling more energized can have an empowering effect on mood and self esteem. The majority of people end up feeling better about themselves (higher self worth) and more in control of their lives (making better decisions) or at least their bodies, especially when they are doing something to improve their health. When one feels more worthy, it is common for libido to increase because they feel more desirable. The benefits of exercise do not stop here either. Not only can it help increase your sex drive, but when you do take part in sex as a fit and healthy person, you will have more stamina in all muscles. This includes the core muscles that may help in some "positions" and provide a better overall experience. One study found that after 9 months on a regular exercise program, the participants not only reported more frequent sexual activity, but they also reported having more satisfying orgasms *(University of California San Diego)*. The reason this can occur in both men and women is that the heart becomes stronger with exercise. Aerobic exercise stimulates the walls of the heart to become thicker and stronger, thereby enabling the heart to pump blood to the rest of the body more efficiently. The number and size of vessels throughout the body also increase, allowing a greater blood supply to be delivered to all tissues. This includes one very important area for men.

Note: I'm not an expert in sexual dysfunction and am not suggesting that exercise alone is the absolute cure for sexual dysfunction, but most experts in this field recommend exercise for these very reasons.

So what happens, sexually, if you do not exercise regularly? A recent article in the Associated Press about a study at the Harvard School of Public Health specifically stated that exercise benefits the small arteries that control erections as well as those that feed the heart. If you do not take care of yourself and these vessels, they will not function as they should. A quote from the very same article suggested, "Maybe the penis is like a barometer of what could happen to your heart and to your brain for stroke" (Dr. William Steers). Dr. Irwin Goldstein commented that studies show that 80% of those who have heart attacks had erectile dysfunction before their attacks. There are several studies showing that the risk of erectile dysfunction drops significantly as exercise increases. In fact, obesity and smoking are probably the two biggest factors that cause impotence. As a man's waist size increases from 32 to 42, his chance of developing erectile dysfunction doubles. If that is not enough motivation to help someone improve their lifestyle, I don't know what is. This does not only apply to men. For women too, you might as well forget about all the benefits discussed above if you're not following the whole plan.

Option 2—For the nights you are not using option 1, or for anyone who does not agree with option 1, there are several things you can do. The point is to keep you from sitting on the couch (all night) eating snacks. If do not have any yoga or Pilates exercise videos I would suggest you get some. These are lower intensity workouts which will help improve your flexibility and core strength. Yoga can also have some additional mental and spiritual benefits that you do not need a tape for. You could also just meditate and clear your mind or gather your thoughts to be prepared for the next day. The choice is yours.

Over the years I have come to realize that not enough people are getting the message about how to take care of themselves. Most of the people I work with have a busy and hectic work and family schedule. Most of us do. Despite our lifestyles it is possible to improve your health and manage your schedule. It comes down to simplifying your life into 3 categories. Self, family, and work. Everything will fall into these three categories, you need to prioritize them and take action so you do not become or continue to be like the Average American.

Chapter 4

Average American
(Keeping the diet industry in business)

Chapter Highlights:

* Obesity is the result of the average American's lifestyle.

* Obesity related diseases and the financial cost of obesity.

* The Super Market Tour

The best of the worst, the worst of the best. It's not such a good thing to be if you know what the statistics are. The average American diet is destroying the health of the average American. The surgeon general reports that 61% of adults and 31% of children in America are considered overweight or obese. According to the *American Obesity Association*, approximately 64.5% of Americans or 127 million adults are overweight. 60 million of them are obese, and 9 million are severely obese. Take a look at the table below which shows the increase in percentage of overweight and obese adults over the past 25 years.

Increase in Prevalence (%) of Overweight (BMI >25),
Obesity (BMI >30) and Severe Obesity (BMI >40) Among U.S. Adults.

	Overweight (BMI >25)	Obesity (BMI >30)	Severe Obesity (BMI >40)
1999 to 2000	64.5	30.5	4.7
1988 to 1994	56.0	23.0	2.9
1976 to 1980	46.0	14.4	No Data

Source: CDC, National Center for Health Statistics, National Health and Nutrition
Examination Survey. Health, United States, 2002. Flegal et. Al. JAMA. 2002;288:1723-7.
NIH, National Heart, Lung, and Blood Institute, Clinical Guidelines on the Identification,
Evaluation and Treatment of Overweight and Obesity in Adults, 1998.

So what exactly is all of this weight gain doing to the average American?

The following is also from the AOA.

Obesity increases the risk of illness from about 30 serious medical conditions.
Obesity is associated with increases in deaths from all causes.
Earlier onset of obesity-related diseases such as type 2 diabetes is being reported in children and adolescents with obesity.
Obesity causes at least 300,000 deaths in the U.S. each year.
The cost of providing health care to obese adults is $100 billion and rising.

Oddly enough, Americans spend about $100 billion on fast food each year. Research shows the average American eats approximately 300 fast food meals each year. All this garbage going in, combined with a lack of activity is resulting in a dramatic shift in the overall health of this country. Even politicians are taking notice of these facts. They understand what it is costing all of us and are looking for alternative ways to pay for it. In New York a 1 percent tax on junk food was proposed to create a pool of money to fight the epidemic of child obesity. A California legislator proposed a 1 cent tax on soda. Why do they believe we should tax these types of products? For the same reason we already feel it is ok to tax cigarettes and alcohol. We know they contribute to long term health problems which cost us all a lot of money. In fact cigarettes only cost the health-care system $75 billion per year compared to today's $117 billion for obesity. The real question is why haven't we done something about this already?

The following is a summary of a study that shows a detailed breakdown on the economic cost of obesity in the U.S.

Current estimates of the economic cost of obesity in the United States
AM Wolf and GA Colditz

The Women's Place, Univ. of Virginia Health Systems, Charlottesville, USA.

This study was undertaken to update and revise the estimate of the economic impact of obesity in the United States. A prevalence-based approach to the cost of illness was used to estimate the economic costs in 1995 dollars attributable to obesity for type 2 diabetes mellitus, coronary heart disease (CHD), hypertension, gallbladder disease, breast, endometrial and colon cancer, and osteoarthritis. Additionally and independently, excess

> *physician visits, work days lost, restricted activity, and bed-days attributable to obesity were analyzed cross-sectionally using the 1998 and 1994 National Health Interview Survey. Direct and indirect costs are from published reports and inflated to 1995 dollars using the medical component of the consumer price index (CPI). The total cost attributable to obesity amounted to $99.2 billion dollars in 1995. Approximately $51.64 billion of those dollars were direct medical costs. Cost of lost productivity attributed to obesity was $3.9 billion and reflected 39.2 million days of lost work.*

The worst or best part about this, depending on how you look at it, is that most of it is preventable. We can combat lifestyle related diseases by "simply" improving our lifestyle. These are not minor diseases either, take a look at the following list and see if you think it might be worth your while to take preventative action.

This is a list of the medical conditions related to obesity:

Osteoarthritis	*Impaired immune Response*
Rheumatoid Arthritis	*Impaired Respiratory Function*
Birth defects	*Infections following wounds*
Cancer	*Infertility*
Cardiovascular disease	*Liver Disease*
Carpel Tunnel Syndrome	*Low back pain*
Chronic Venous insufficiency	*Obstetric and Gynecologic complications*
Daytime Sleepiness	*Pain*
Deep Vein Thrombosis (DVT)	*Pancreatitis*
Diabetes Type 2	*Sleep Apnea*
Gout	*Stroke*
Heat Disorders	*Surgical Complications*
Hypertension	*Urinary Stress Incontinence*

How and why are so many Americans allowing this to happen?

The following chart from AOA shows how modernization of society's impact of the health of the average American.

Location or Type of Activity	Effect of Modernization	Impact on Obesity
Transportation	Rise in car ownership. Increase in driving shorter distances.	Decrease in walking or cycling
At Home	Increase in the use of modern appliances (e.g. microwaves, dishwashers, washing machines, vacuum cleaners Increase in ready-made foods and ingredients for cooking. Increase in television viewing, and computer and video game use.	Decrease in manual labor Increase in consumption of convenience foods that contribute to obesity. Decrease in time spent on more active recreational pursuits.
In the Work Place	Increase in sedentary occupational lifestyles due to technology— increase in computerization.	Decrease in physically demanding manual labor.
Public Places	Increase in use of elevators, escalators and automatic doors.	Decrease in daily physical activity patterns such as climbing stairs.
Urban Residency	Increase in crime in urban areas.	Prevents women, children and elderly from going out alone for exercise and leisure activities.

The one area that probably effects Americans more than any other is the at home section. This is also the one area we have the most control over. The increase in modern appliances should have freed up more time for us, so the decrease in manual labor becomes a non-issue. The real issue is how we use that extra time. Unfortunately for many it is spent sitting in front of the TV or their computer. The health experts have been saying we are becoming a nation of couch potatoes for awhile now, but you'll never imagine how bad it really has become. There was an article written by AP writer Daniel Yee (Aug 14, 03) about a study recently conducted by The Centers for Disease Control and Prevention. The following contains a few selections from this article.

> **"Despite broader exercise definition, most Americans still don't get enough"**
> *Even when sweeping, waiting tables and tossing a Frisbee count as exercise, most Americans still aren't getting enough of it.*
>
> *The Centers for Disease Control and Prevention, believing earlier studies failed to accurately measure Americans' fitness because they focused on intense exercise, has lumped everyday activities such as housework and gardening with jogging and lifting weights.*
>
> *But even with playing with children and raking the lawn on the list of moderate-intensity activities, the 2001 phone survey released Thursday showed that 55 percent of adults still didn't get the recommended minimum: 30 minutes a day, at least four days a week.*
>
> *"It's surprising," said Harold Kohl of the CDC, who authored the study. "There's still more than one out of two Americans who are not active at a level we think promotes health…we've really got to move the needle substantially from where it is right now."*
>
> *The recommendations are just the minimums to prevent people from developing chronic diseases such as high blood pressure or diabetes. The Institute of Medicine says people should double the CDC's recommendations—60 minutes of moderate exercise a day—to drop pounds. (Daniel Yee, AP Writer, Thur Aug 12 2003)*

The writer goes on to state that, health officials say Americans' lack of exercise is one of the nations most pressing health problems. We really need to get out more and do the recreational activities we enjoy. If you can't do that, go and get some equipment from a local fitness dealer so you can workout in your home. If you need to be in front of the TV, you can at least watch it while you are on the treadmill. There really should not be any excuses. For those who say, "I can't afford it", you really can't afford not to do it. Wait until you see the amount of money it will cost you when your health goes downhill. Take a look at these numbers for *Prudential Life insurance* ™ underwriting classifications. Insurers use these classifications to set premium rates based on your health and lifestyle. The scoring system looks at your blood pressure, medical conditions, and driving record. The following is for a 35 year old man (in good health) seeking a $500,000 10 year level premium term.

Category	Annual Rate
Preferred Best	$335
Preferred Plus	$380
Preferred Nonsmoker	$440
Nonsmoker	$520
Preferred Plus Smoker	$875
Smoker	$1,120 *(Star-Ledger, Dec 3, 00 sec 3 p 1)*

If you are a nonsmoker who happens to be overweight and out of shape you will probably have more medical conditions than just high blood pressure. Without even considering the additional costs of health insurance, medications and more doctor visits, you will pay up to 40% more just for a life insurance policy and that's if they even accept you. Insurance companies will sometimes turn you down completely if they feel you are too much of a risk.

The next major issue from the modernization chart is the increase in consumption of convenience foods. This is one of my major areas of focus with new clients. During their first few weeks of their program they go through a supermarket education tour. This teaches the individual to understand how to read food labels so they truly know what is in the foods they are buying. The first part of the tour covers the overall layout of the store. The fresh foods, produce, meat, dairy, and seafood are all along the store perimeter. This is where you want to get most of your foods from. Next we get into a three step lesson plan.

Lesson one of the tour points out the fact that most of the isles are filled with boxed or canned convenience foods. These convenience foods are usually filled with preservatives, sodium, hydrogenated oils (Trans Fats), refined sugars, and all the ingredients to destroy your health. Some of these ingredients increase the foods shelf life, so the manufacturer has a better chance of selling it before it spoils. This helps increase profits (Now that's convenient). This is not to say that every item in a box or can is bad, old-fashioned oatmeal is one such exception, but you are usually better off avoiding most convenience foods. One other note on this topic is cost. Many have the misconception that eating healthy is more expensive. This is not always the case; in fact most times you can save money by avoiding the pre-packaged convenience foods. Foods in their natural form are not only healthier for you but you are not paying for packaging and materials. Whenever someone makes anything more convenient for you, there is always a premium for that.

Lesson two covers the reading of food labels and understanding macronutrients. Carbohydrates and proteins have a caloric value of approximately 4 calories per gram, while fats are 9 calories per gram. As you can see fats have more than twice the amount of calories for the same serving size. This is why one should limit their fat intake. However, that is not to say all fats are bad or that you should restrict fat intake altogether. There are many sources of good fats which you need in your diet. We will cover this topic in more detail in the nutrition chapter. For now this knowledge will educate you about what is actually in the foods you consume. Many of my clients are quite surprised when they see examples of everyday foods and how they break down.

One such example is the label on 1% milk: (summary of actual label)

Nutrition Facts		
serving size 1 cup (240ml)		
Servings per container About 16		
Amount Per Serving		
Calories 100	Fat Cal. 20	
% Daily Value		
Total Fat 2.5 g		4%
Saturated fat 1.5 g		
Total Carb. 12 g		4%
Sugars 12 g		
Protein 8 g		16%

1 serving of 1% milk (1 cup) is 100 calories, 12 grams of carbohydrate, 8 grams of protein, and 2.5 grams of fat. If we calculate that out, 2.5 grams of fat X 9 calories per gram, we see that 22.5 of the 100 calories come from fat. If we take those 22.5 calories and divide by 100, we see that 22.5%, not 1% of the calories come from fat. Now this does not necessitate drinking skim milk, but people need to understand what they are getting. The fat in milk is measured by volume, not by calories like most people would think. The same applies to ground meat. Next time you go shopping, look at the label of ground beef, chicken, or turkey.

(Summary of actual label)

Nutrition Facts
serving size 4oz (112g)
Servings per container varies

Amount Per Serving		
Calories 240 Fat Cal. 150		

% Daily Value		
Total Fat 17 g		26%
Saturated fat 4.5 g		

Total Carb. 0 g		0%
Sugars 0 g		

Protein 20 g		

This was the information directly off of an 85% lean turkey package. As you can see, on a serving size of approximately 240 calories, 150 calories come from fat. That is over 50%. This is because, like milk, the percentage of fat in meat is not measured by calories. Most people do not realize this. Anyone trying to limit their fat intake should buy the leaner (97–99% lean) cuts of meat. When you do the math you will see they still have a fair amount of fat in them, just make sure you do not over cook them or you will dry them out.

The next step in improving your health depends upon the choices you make regarding the quality of the foods you eat. There are many different levels you can take your program to; how far you go is up to you. Bread is one such level. This can vary greatly from brand to brand, but rye bread generally has the lowest calorie, carb, and sugar count of all the types of bread. It has approximately 80 calories per slice, with 16–18 grams of carbs and 1–2 grams of sugar. Next is oat bran, with 100, 18–20, and 2–3, followed by whole-wheat with 110, 20–24, and 6. Most of us know the reasons we should avoid the highly processed white breads, but there is no reason a healthy active adult cannot consume these other breads. With all the "Low Carb" products coming out these days, it's beginning to seem like the "Fat Free" & "Sugar Free" days all over again. Just about everyone missed the point back then, and they are missing the point now. All that stuff is not "calorie free". Another area or level has to do with fish. You may have seen reports over the past few years on the dangers of shark, swordfish, tile fish, and tuna. The levels of pollutants can be especially dangerous for pregnant women and the fetus. Eat enough of these and I'm sure it could be harmful to most people, but this does not mean that all fish are bad. One last topic I always cover with my clients is red meat. If you are going to eat red meat, eat grass fed, organic, free range beef. Most industrial farm cattle are fed with grains, pumped with antibiotics and growth hormones and fattened up before slaughter to earn top dollar. You can read from hundreds of articles and books on the benefits of organic foods and farming practices. Over the past few years more and more health and fitness professionals are taking this path. For expert opinions on this matter check out Dr. Joseph Mercola's website at mercola.com or read his book: The No Grain Diet. For a quick guide to understanding the difference between industrial farming and organic, the following are excerpts from an article by Paul Chek.

"Dr. Price found that healthy populations who farmed their food used organic farming principles. These cultures always used a natural cycle of returning animal and vegetable wastes to the soil, which made for healthy soils, plants, animals and ultimately, healthy people. This is almost completely opposite to the situation we have today. Poor farming practices under the seductive influence of chemical corporations have left us with millions of acres of damaged, mineral-depleted soils. Such disrespectful farming practices and abuse of agrochemicals have served to benefit medical establishments, veterinary medicine and the drug companies that supply them, while progressively making humanity sick and diseased. As the vitality of humans and animals declines due to chemical farming methods and disrespect for the soil, the incidence of many human diseases, particularly cancers and degenerative diseases is skyrocketing at an alarming rate.

How many people today even stop to question where the food they are eating came from? People don't seem to care what's in their food, what the 15-syllable ingredients mean, what synthetic chemicals were added, what was sprayed on their food to protect it from pests or what colors were added to make it look better! While some $110 billion is spent each year on fast food in the US, we treat food like it is just another commodity you can pick up at the local store. All the while, we are becoming more ignorant to the fact that the foods we are eating may be the most toxic substances we come in contact with all day, yet some people eat fast food all three meals!

Commercially grown produce and commercially raised meat are two big reasons disease is so rampant in our society. Today's crops are sprayed with unfathomable amounts of chemicals, pesticides, fungicides and herbicides, not to mention the soil crops are grown in is devoid of any nutrients. Commercially raised meat is no better. These animals are raised in unsanitary conditions, are forced to consume things they were never designed to eat (i.e., cement, cardboard and other animal remains) and injected full of antibiotics just to keep them alive because they are so diseased." (Personal Fitness Professional July 03, p20–21)

Lesson Three covers the topic of understanding what is in nutritional supplements. Here is a great quote regarding the use of supplements, "we are trying to fine tune our metabolic engines, when they are not even firing on all cylinders" (anonymous). If you can make it through your day on regular whole foods alone, you will probably be better off. Not many can argue with the fact that we need more whole foods, fruits, and vegetables in our diet, or that if we did eat them, we could improve many of the current health issues. However, if your schedule does not allow for you to plan all your meals, supplements can be of great value to fill in the nutritional gaps in your day.

There are many products out there to choose from. The sale of supplements has grown into a $15 billion industry. Unfortunately some companies are just trying to jump on the supplement bandwagon to increase sales. This creates a situation where not all supplements are of high quality and some are designed for very specific purposes which may not match your nutritional needs. It can make it very confusing for one to find the right product. See the supplements section in appendix VII to gain a better understanding of the products on the market. The key to using supplements properly is to know what makes one product better than another. The supermarket tour covers this topic using examples of both good and poor choices as you will discover in the following sections.

One such comparison is *SlimFast* ™vs. *Chips A'hoy*™:

1 Serving of a SlimFast meal replacement shake contains 220 calories
40 grams of carbohydrate (35 of which come directly from refined sugar)
10 grams of protein
2.5 grams of fat
The most significant number there is the sugar. That is a ridiculous amount of sugar contained in a product that is advertised to help you lose weight and improve your health. If you have diabetes or are at all concerned about it, you may be better off just eating an equal serving size of cookies along with a multi-vitamin.

4 Chips A'hoy cookies contain 213 calories
28 grams of carbohydrate (13 from sugar)
2.6 grams of protein
10.6 grams of fat

As you can see the cookies have far less sugar and therefore will cause less of a spike in your blood sugar levels. When you ingest a sugary snack, your blood sugar level spikes up and the pancreas must pump out insulin to bring sugar levels back down. Over time with regular and frequent occurrences, this insulin response can stress the pancreas and contribute to diabetes. Also when insulin levels are increased, fat storage also increases. Although these cookies will cause less of a spike than the SlimFast, they are still cookies, so do not think that they are acceptable as a supplement. The point of this lesson is to help everyone realize how important it is to read the labels and not just grab any bar or shake off the shelf. Since writing this example, *Slimfast* ™ has created a new formulation to join the low carb frenzy. However, this new formula still contains 19–24 grams of sugar per serving. Food manufacturers are like surfers looking for the next big wave. They don't have a care in the world (for your health) as long as they can catch (your money) the next big wave. Remember that and you might start looking at packaged foods differently.

Now that we understand not all products are high quality, the question is; how do you find the good ones? Typically, protein powders for shakes are of higher quality than bars for several reasons. Bars usually have some additional ingredients to make them more palatable, i.e., taste, texture…Many times this can bring down the nutritional quality. However, since bars are very popular we will cover a few of the more well known ones. If you are going to compete in some type of event (biking, hiking, etc.) and you want a burst of energy for that period of time you would want to select an energy type bar. *Clif Bars*™ and *Power Bars* ™ are two good choices in that category. Both of these bars have a higher concentration of simple and complex carbohydrates to give you an energy burst. If you are looking for something to replace a meal or as a balanced snack, you want a bar that is more balanced in macronutrients. Two common choices are *Balance Bars*™, and *Zone Bars*™. These two bars are decent in quality and taste, although there are some higher quality bars out there. If this is more your goal you should select a bar to your liking that meets the following criteria. **First**, try to keep the sugars under 10 grams or at least no more than half of the total carbohydrate content. **Second**, keep the protein grams higher than the total sugar content. Look for a range of 10–30 grams of protein. **Third,** read the overall ingredient label to look for red flags. The protein source, for instance, usually whey protein isolate or concentrate, soy protein, casein, and milk protein are all good sources. If you see the words like hydrolyzed collagen or gelatin, these are cheap low quality sources of protein and you should look for another bar. For a list of bars that meet this criteria see insert:

List of bars that meet criteria:

Myoplex Lite™ - 180 calories, 26g of carbs (12 sugar), 4.5g of fat, 15g of protein
Nitro-Tech™   - 300 calories, 6g of carbs (2g sugar), 8g of fat, 35g of protein
Parillo Bar™   - 240 calories, 35g of carbs (3g sugar), 6g of fat, 14g of protein
Zone Perfect™ - 190 calories, 21g of carbs (12 sugar), 7g of fat, 16g of protein

Note: There are others out there as well, use these as a reference. Some of these are borderline on making the grade, pay attention to different flavors from the same company which may not make the cut.

Armed with this information on the foods you are putting into your body, you now at least have the knowledge to make better decisions. The next chapter will help you to better grasp the concept of creating a balanced nutrition plan and your actual menu.

Chapter 5

Nutrition

Chapter Highlights:

- How to balance your food intake and why carbohydrates are an important component.

- Calories in vs. calories out, and calculating your resting metabolic rate (RMR).

- Maintaining your progress, what to do when you have reached your goal.

- Water

First and foremost, we need to get something absolutely clear—There is a difference between a "diet" and a lifelong weight maintenance program. A diet is something that many people have tried, over and over, and failed to maintain the results they attained while on the program. The reason is simple; it is not possible to stay on many of these plans for the rest of your life. A weight maintenance program is different. Think of anything that needs regular maintenance i.e. your computer, your car, your house etc. If you do not take care of these things on a regular basis something can go wrong. Your body is a machine that needs regular maintenance in much the same way. Unfortunately most people do not see it this way and they neglect to take care of it. Compounding the problem further, most people are reluctant to spend money on taking care of their health. Many people hold back on going to the dentist, doctor, hiring a personal trainer, or even spending a little extra on the purchase of quality exercise equipment. Some do not think they need the help, while others are in denial. Either way, they do not see the value in maintaining a healthy body, yet they wouldn't think twice about getting an oil change, brake overhaul, or even getting a new furnace. All these things over the course of a year can add up to thousands of dollars, but is any of that more important than your health? You may be able to get a new car every few years if you grow tired of your current one, but you will always be stuck with the same body—Take care of it.

Ok, let's get back to the topic, defining a lifelong weight maintenance program and how it is different from a diet. In a weight maintenance program, nutrition is only a part of the entire program. When used in combination with exercise and rest, you can get results that are maintainable. Unlike in some of the more popular diets out there, carbohydrates can and should be included as part of a balanced intake of nutrients. We will get into the details of this with the Steady Pace plan later in this chapter. For those of you who may be thinking "well if I eat carbs I just know I won't lose weight", you are wrong. You may not lose 10 lbs in two weeks; however, the weight you lose can be maintained.

There are two basic plans for weight loss. The first is for all those out there who fear the word "CARBS"; they label themselves as a carb addict and feel they may be out of control with their eating. People in this category may have frequent cravings, or weight related health issues. They may want to get a jump start on their weight loss effort. Thus, the name of this first plan is "Jump Start". It is an initial phase that can last anywhere from 3 to 14 days. We are all somewhat familiar with the Atkins approach, and by now should understand that it is not the healthiest of options. We have also learned that due to the nature of the plan much of the weight lost on Atkins is not from fat and is therefore not permanent. There are some very similar types of diets out there, some of which take a more sensible and healthier approach. They stress the importance of eating leaner meats and fish as well as an adequate intake of healthy fats. Many individuals have experienced great initial results on these plans and they have become extremely popular. Some, you may have heard of and some you may not. Two such diets are the *South Beach Diet*, and the *No Grain Diet*. You may wonder why I would reveal the names of any such plan that might compete with my own program. However, these diets are not revealing any special secrets. In fact similar plans have been around for quite a long time now. These plans in some ways are actually quite similar to what I do with some of my own clients.

The Jump Start phase takes you off of nearly all simple carbohydrates including most grains, starches, and sugary snacks. This "cold turkey" approach allows your body to avoid the dramatic insulin reactions we discussed in the supermarket tour. Some claim this helps your body to lose its addiction and cravings for unhealthy foods and allows it to adjust to more wholesome foods. Just as withdrawal from an addictive drug can affect the body physically and psychologically, there can be a variety of reactions as one moves from empty nutrition to a whole foods diet filled with vitamins, minerals and fiber. There probably is some truth to this matter. More and more studies are coming out which demonstrate how sugar, and sugary snacks can be addictive. Many of my own clients have commented about how they found they did not enjoy eating some of these foods after being off of them for awhile. In fact some claimed it upset their stomach after eating sweets or fatty foods.

In the No Grain Diet, Dr. Mercola advises starting the diet on a Friday so you have the weekend to adjust to the plan. I agree with this idea, unless of course you have a busy Friday, then Saturday would make more sense. The point being, select a two day period when you will have enough time to plan it all out and see what works and what does not. Once you learn how to plan meals and prepare foods ahead of time, you will be ready to do what it takes entering your first full week on the plan. Let's say for example, you are someone who is short on time. You must come up with techniques to help you save time and be successful. For instance, if you do not have time to prepare dinner every night of the week, you should cook excess portions on the nights you can. This way you can freeze the leftovers and reheat them for a quick and easy meal on your busy nights. As I tell my clients, you can always take things as far as you feel is necessary for you to be successful. If you want to take this example a step further, you can freeze the food into pre-measured, separate containers to make it that much easier when you do need them. Another great way to save time is with breakfast. Many Sunday nights, I will hard boil 12–18 eggs, so that I can simply peel and eat them over the following few mornings rather than take the time to cook eggs each morning.

A sample meal planner for all phases of your program is provided in appendix I & II. The key to following the plan once you have all the food you need in your house and none of the food you don't, is to document your food intake. Journaling your food intake is an extremely important part of planning your daily meals. It makes you more aware of the type and amount of food you are putting into your body and it allows you to review your intake and make any necessary improvements. You can use any notebook for this. When you begin your program, you will be eating every 2–3 hours for a total of 4–6 meals per day. This will do several things for you. **First**, if you eat small balanced meals throughout the day, your blood sugar levels will be more consistent. This will reduce hunger pangs, cravings, and keep energy levels more consistent. **Second**, if you eat every few hours you really won't have enough time between meals to get extremely hungry.

Many times I have a new client tell me during their initial interview that they are usually very hungry come dinner time. It turns out these are the same people who don't eat much during the day. **Third**, every time you eat, your body has to digest the food. The digestion process itself, requires energy and you will actually burn calories. This is called the Thermic Effect of food (TEF). Complex carbohydrates and proteins have a higher TEF while simple carbs and fats have a low effect. For example if you were to eat 100 calories of a high TEF food 15 calories may be burned up in the digestion process and you would only net 85 calories. On the other hand, with a low TEF food you may net 95 of 100 calories. This is why it is so important to eat high quality foods.

While Jump Start can be a great way to get your program started, it is not always necessary or optimal for all individuals. For any critics out there who would question why I would even suggest an initial "low carb" phase like jump start, the reason is that I have worked with enough people on these types of diets to see that they can maintain their results as they transition to a more balanced food intake combined with exercise.

There is a second option for those who are more in control and need some help putting a sound plan together and making better choices. Many of my clients have been very successful with their programs by simply making better choices and planning their meals. It is usually best to make several small, but significant changes that are easy to maintain. Several small modifications can have a large cumulative effect on one's health. This also results in a plan that is not drastically different from one's current eating habits and they therefore feel more capable of following it, thus creating a permanent lifestyle change. This second path is called the "Steady Pace" plan. If you feel capable of skipping the cold turkey approach, than you should begin with the Steady Pace plan. However, if you feel you need to make a dramatic change to break old habits Jump Start is for you.

When someone starts out on the Steady Pace they are also going to eat small balanced meals throughout the day in the same manner as Jump Start. They will also get all the same benefits already mentioned. Steady Pace also requires that you avoid <u>refined</u> grains, starches and sugars. The difference is, with the exception of the last one or two meals of the day, you can and should eat more high quality complex carbohydrates, i.e. whole grains. These are part of a balanced intake that helps to give you the energy to live an active lifestyle. This balance is especially important when you are involved in an exercise program. If you were to stay on a low carbohydrate diet for too long, your energy levels will drop. Physical lethargy is not the only side effect. Mental "slowness" will also occur since carbohydrates are the preferred fuel source for the brain. Low carb diet gurus sometimes fail to mention these side effects and the true importance of carbohydrates. The Steady Pace plan has a significant advantage of over the Jump Start plan because of this balance and will therefore provide you with more energy. Increasing our energy levels is a big part of improving our health, and having enough energy to take on an exercise program is a big part of my plan. As you will learn in the following chapters, I do not just suggest you get involved in an exercise program. I explain the details about the fact that you MUST get involved in an exercise program if you want to create a permanent change. This is an important factor in why this program will work.

Believe it or not, nutrition in many ways is fairly simple; it's about creating a calorie deficit. What it all comes down to is a fairly simple formula. It's a matter of calories in vs. calories out. What can be a little more complex is when you are actually eating those calories and what the quality of those calories is. The menu guidelines provided in the appendix will help to steer you in the right direction. To shed some light on this subject I refer you to the story of Pam as well as some menu examples.

When Pam first came to me she was on her last string of hope. She had tried everything out there; she was a fad diet expert. She had lost and gained more weight than she could count and was frustrated with herself, past programs, and the results she got from them. During our first interview she became upset because she was already envisioning a future failure. Once she realized I knew what she was feeling and she saw my confidence in being able to help her, a little light turned on. We slowly began a process of changing some of her past beliefs that had led her to take her past actions.

Pam came to me at 184 pounds, 48 years old and inexperienced with regards to a sound exercise program, especially weight training. Like most women she had tried a few classes that used light hand weights and never really got results from it. She did however do a walking routine regularly, 3–4 days per week. Her food intake, on the surface, was very little. She reported that she mostly skipped breakfast, maybe had coffee or orange juice. Lunch was noodle soup and a diet soda; she snacked on candy or chips in the afternoon and had a chicken salad for dinner. She also had ice cream about 3 nights per week.

You might think that is not much food and she should be fine with that amount. However, the first problem with people who "don't eat that much" is that they are only aware of a portion of their total calories. Whether they truly don't realize what they are doing or they just cannot admit it to themselves, they are eating more calories. If you really want to make a permanent change, you need to be totally honest with yourself and face reality. Another major problem is the fact that Pam reported she mostly skips breakfast. Any time you skip breakfast you set yourself up for a slower start to your metabolism each day you do it. It delays the process of your body turning on and burning calories. One thing is for sure, it may not make sense to you, but it is very difficult to lose weight if you are going to skip breakfast. The main problem with Pam's style of eating is that when someone tries to eat "light" during the day they end up eating more in the evening. Your body needs a certain amount of calories and you will eventually have to eat them no matter how hard you try to fight it.

The next problem looking at Pam's food intake was the quality of the actual foods she was eating. If it wasn't for the chicken on her salad for dinner, her day was virtually void of any protein. If you want to get lean and fit, you need to have a decent amount of protein in your diet. In fact just about all meals should be balanced in terms of containing protein, carbohydrate, and fats. This is the essence of my program. You see, just about anyone out there could use a little fine-tuning to their diet to improve their chance for results, and that is what I do. I first take a look at what someone is currently doing and then I decide how to improve upon that. So when I see a breakfast skipper with low protein intake, I know there is plenty of room for improvement. One point I must make absolutely clear, I am not a dietician and I do not design specific menu plans for anyone. What I do, is educate people on what certain foods will do for your body and how to make the right choices to balance their intake. Before you start thinking, "what does this guy know, he's not even a dietician or a doctor", let me answer a few questions and state the facts.

Do I have a background in nutrition? Yes, part of my undergraduate and graduate education involved courses in nutrition for sports performance as well as diet and weight loss. I have also been working in this field for nine years now.

Are my clients successful? Yes, in nine years I have only had one client, who claimed to be following their program, not lose weight.

Just because a trainer is not a licensed dietician does not mean they cannot guide you towards the path of better health and fitness. In fact, many times physicians and dieticians come to trainers like me because they need help losing weight.

Your first step to fine-tuning your own diet is to journal your food intake and compare it to the menu guidelines. The food selections within these guidelines are merely examples of things you can eat. If I listed broccoli with a particular meal and you do not like it, feel free to eat asparagus instead. These examples are intended to show you what a balanced meal looks like. If you happen to like any or all of the meals I have listed, then you can choose to eat them as they are. When you do get started on your plan, stick with it. You must give it at least a week or two to see how your body reacts to it. Sometimes people get bored quickly and want to make adjustments to their plan before they even give it a chance to work. This will not get you anywhere. I have trained clients who were so carbohydrate depleted that when they began their plan and actually ate some quality carbohydrates their body soaked them up along with water. In some cases they gained 1 or 2 pounds in the first week. This can be frustrating if one does not know what is actually happening. Those who followed my advice and stuck with their plan lost 1–2 pounds from their original weight at the end of 3 weeks. More importantly they lost inches, body fat and felt great once they learned what was happening. Remember, losing body fat while feeding the muscle to support the metabolism is what you want to do. The scale alone should not be your guide and should never determine how you feel about yourself.

> *Note: If for any reason after three weeks you can honestly say that you followed your entire program, put in 100% effort and did not notice any changes, you may want to get your thyroid tested.*

Let's get started with what you should do on the first day of your program. To balance out your breakfast start with a good protein source. Proteins are used to build muscle tissue, are a major component of key enzymes, and can serve as an energy source when needed. Proteins are made up of carbon, oxygen, hydrogen, and nitrogen which help to form amino acids. Our bodies use 20 amino acids, some of which the body can make on its own, others need to be taken in through our diet. Lean cuts of meat, poultry, fish, and game animals are good quality protein sources, dairy products and plant foods also contain protein. For breakfast, eggs are a popular choice; organic eggs would be a better choice. Now cook them however you like, but keep your ratio of whites to yolks at 3:1. One egg white is approximately 20 calories and 5 grams of protein. One whole egg is approximately 70 calories the extra 50 calories coming mostly from fat in the yolk. So you can see that 3 whites and one yolk will yield approximately 110 calories and 15–18 grams of protein. 15–30 grams per meal and 4–6 meals per day will keep you on pace to take in 1–1.5 grams of protein per pound of lean body weight. There are a wide range of recommendations here; I tend to stay closer to the low end of this one in most cases. Another more commonly used rule is 1–2 grams per kilogram of body weight. Either of these should keep you in a safe and effective range. However, you do not want to exceed either of these ranges because your body cannot really handle doses of more than 30 grams per meal, nor can it handle excess amounts over the course of a day. If you exceed these amounts, your body will convert some of it to fat and excrete some of it as urea. Over time this may put stress on the liver and the kidneys since the liver is the main organ involved in protein metabolism and the kidneys convert excess nitrogen into urea.

For calculating your appropriate amount, the equations below will assist you:

Example 1—your lean body weight is your lean mass. If you have ever had your body fat measured, you know what this is. If you have not, the following example should help you to understand.

If Tammy goes down to the local health club to get her body fat measured and it turns out to be 20%. She is in the healthy category which ranges from 20–26% for men and up to 33% for women. According to the statistics, most Americans are above this level. Now if Tammy weighs 100 lbs, that means her lean mass is 80 pounds and she has 20 pounds of fat. To calculate her protein intake we can take 80 X 1–1.5 and get a range of 80–120 grams of protein.

Example 2—divide your weight in pounds by 2.2, this equals your weight in kilograms. Multiply this number by 1–2 and you have your recommended grams per day.

Next we need a carbohydrate source. These are the foods that give you energy and add fiber into your diet. Fruits and vegetables, beans and legumes, oats, Oatmeal is always a great choice. As I mentioned in chapter 4, there are always levels of quality with foods. Oatmeal has several. Steel cut and Irish oats can take nearly an hour to cook. Next is whole grain oats, then quick oats, and finally microwave packets with flavors. The longer it takes to cook, the longer it takes your body to break it down and the better it is for you. One serving (1/2 cup) is 150 calories. Oatmeal has a high fiber content and low glycemic index which will help to slow the digestion of your meal and diminishes the blood sugar/insulin response that typically occurs with carbohydrate ingestion. This will result in you feeling full and satisfied longer after a meal. One last thing to finish off this meal is to add some fruit, throw some blueberries in the oatmeal. Some "low carb" gurus want you to nearly eliminate fruit because of the sugar content. This eliminates some great nutrients, you may be better off by limiting your intake to two servings early in the day and get a variety of fruits, especially berries.

As far as fat is concerned, you do not need to look too hard to get fat into your diet. Many items you eat are going to give you more fat than you need as you already learned from the Super Market Tour. The problem is the type of fat you want is not usually what you get. For example in the breakfast above, you are getting fat from the egg yolk, and depending on what you cooked them in (butter, Pam, bacon grease), you probably got more. A good portion of this fat is saturated fat; many animal sources contain the saturated fats which you do not necessarily need, especially in excess. Most plants contain the essential fats you do want. Think olives (olive oil), nuts (almonds, walnuts), seeds (flaxseeds or flaxseed oil), and fish oils (salmon).You want to make sure you get in the poly and monounsaturated fats, the essential Omega-3 fats are what most people need more of in their diet. According to Dr. Mercola and other experts in this matter, the Omega 6 to Omega 3 ratio in those who consume a high carbohydrate diet is near 12:1, when it should be near 3:1 for optimal health. Most people do not eat enough foods rich in Omega-3 fats. These essential fats are essential because your liver cannot make them and your body needs them. You can get them by eating the foods listed above or by taking supplements for them such as flax seed oil or fish oils. There is even a cereal called Uncle Sam's™ contains flaxseeds. Fats, essential or not, are very beneficial. They are part of virtually all cell membrane structures and are used as insulators and shock absorbers to protect your organs; they are also used for energy.

The breakfast shown below is a good example of how to start a balanced day:

1 whole egg	- 70 calories
2 egg whites	- 40 calories
½ cup oatmeal	- 150 calories
¼ cup blueberries	- 50 calories
TOTAL	= 310 calories

At 4–6 meals per day this would get you to a range of 1200–1800 calories per day. For most people this is enough calories to support a healthy weight loss. The average women's basal or resting metabolic rate (RMR) is approximately

1200–1500 calories, for men it is around 1800 because they naturally have more muscle mass. Again this is for average, not fit individuals whose metabolism may be significantly higher. If you are eating enough calories to be near your base metabolism, any activity you do will create a gap between calories in and calories out. To calculate your RMR, there is a calculator on the internet at **www.room42.com/nutrition/basal.shtml**, this is only an estimation formula, but it can give you an idea of what your RMR is. There are several variables that can cause the numbers to go up or down. Age, body weight, activity levels, and what you may have done to your body in past diets. For the purposes of this book these numbers are a fair estimate of RMR.

If you would like a more accurate measure you can get your metabolism tested. If you are interested you should see if your local health club offers *BODY GEM*™ testing. Whichever method you choose, once you determine the appropriate intake based on your goals, metabolism, and activity levels, you can move on to the next step.

When creating a fat loss plan several factors need to be considered. Depending on the activity level, caloric intake should be near RMR. When combined with exercise, we can create a gap of 500–1000 calories per day. This will equate to a 3500 to7000 calorie gap per week or a fat loss of 1–2 lbs. Some of you who have read some other plans may be thinking, "I don't know if I like this, the other plans said I don't need to count calories". What you need to understand is that most of the plans that make that claim are most likely a low carb plan. They can say this because if you are not eating carbs, it is very difficult to eat enough total calories. The main reason calories and portion sizes need to be accounted for in the beginning is because many people are out of control or have no idea what normal portions sizes are. I have known clients who can eat a basket full of apples in one sitting instead of just one. A huge steak is sometimes a common meal. Many people need to get a sense of what healthy portion sizes are. These days when we go out to eat, many restaurants "Supersize" our portions to win us over. The larger portion sizes make us feel better about the "value" we are getting. At some restaurants these portions are getting way out of control and unfortunately so are their patron's waistlines. You do not need to measure foods and count calories forever; just until you develop an understanding of what is the appropriate amount for your body.

To help you formulate a clear understanding of how to balance meals and calorie intake, the following is a sample of a daily meal plan:

	JUMP START			STEADY PACE	
Meal 1:	1 cup	Uncle Sam's Cereal	1		Banana
	¼ cup	Blueberries	¼ cup		Pineapple
	2	Egg whites	3–4		Strawberries
	1	Whole egg	1 scoop		Protein powder
	1 cup	skim milk	1 cup		Plain yogurt
Meal 2:	1	Apple	1 cup		Kashi Go-Lean
	6 oz	Almonds	1 cup		Cottage Cheese
			¼ cup		Blueberries
Meal 3:	Stir-Fry		1 cup		Brown Rice
	5 oz	Beef or Chicken	1		Chicken Breast
	2 cups	Mixed veggies	1 cup		Broccoli
Meal 4:	3 oz	Tuna	2 oz		Buffalo Jerky
	1 Tbsp	Balsamic vinaigrette	¼ cup		Mixed Nuts
	¼ cup	Diced tomatoes			
Meal 5:	1	Chicken Breast	4–5 oz		Alaskan salmon
	2 cups	Salad greens	2 cups		Mixed veggies
	1 Tbsp	Olive oil & vinegar			
*Meal 6: 1		Protein Shake (milk & protein powder only)	3		Egg whites

Looking at the two examples, you should notice two major points. First, each meal, especially with the steady pace plan, is balanced between carbohydrate, protein, and fat. Second, as the day goes on the starchy carbohydrates were reduced and eventually removed from the last meal. The salad and veggies are both carbohydrates, they just have a lower calorie content and higher nutrient content. Some of you might think you need to have something like rice or pasta or some side dish to help you feel like you are having a complete dinner. The fact is many people who feel this way do not eat enough during the day. Your body needs a certain level of carbohydrate intake; if you can satisfy this need during the day with quality foods you will be just fine with the above type of dinner. If for some reason it is not enough food for you and you need additional calories, that is when meal 6 would be used. This is an optional meal to boost your overall calorie intake and keep you from snacking on any carbohydrates or fats at night. As your metabolism revs up there are two modifications you can make. When you begin to see results, the optional meal becomes a regular meal. You will notice your hunger levels increasing when it is time to incorporate this. Second, once you get to where you want to be (if the goal was weight/fat loss), we can add some quality carbohydrates such as brown rice or sweet potatoes back to the dinner meal. This is the "Maintenance phase" of the plan, where we can add more calories to the daily intake as your metabolism and activity levels increase. The "Maintenance Phase" is a nice place to be considering the fact that when you get there it means you have attained your goal. Acknowledging its existence is knowing you will not be in any of the other phases forever. When I say, you do not have to do a particular phase forever; overall I'm referring to the fact that you do not have to be as regimented with your plan. Once you attain your goal, you will have more freedom of choice with your food. Make no mistake, you must still eat healthy and this is a plan that you can continue for a lifetime. However, if you return to your old habits, you will eventually return to your old body.

Water

There is one last topic that is extremely important, water. There was no mention of fruit juices or sodas (diet or regular) in the sample menu because they have absolutely no place in this plan. If you really want to see results you should be drinking water and maybe some tea, nothing else. Our body is mostly made up of water and there are many benefits to drinking water. There are many recommendations of how much you should drink. Some say you should drink it warm, cold, distilled…The fact that you should drink the cleanest (filtered if necessary) water you can find. As far as how much, 8–10 8oz glasses should do for the average person. Another guideline is .5 X your body wt, or .5 X 200 lbs = 100 oz. If you live in a drier climate or at a higher altitude you may need more, and the more active you are the more you will need. One study from the University of Utah in Salt Lake City demonstrated that subjects drinking only half the recommended water intake experienced a 5% reduction in blood plasma volumes and moderate dehydration. This can lead to symptoms of fatigue, reduced ability to concentrate, and headaches. Why is water so important? It is a part of nearly every function of our bodies.

The benefits of water are as follows:

- Helps regulate body temperature
- Helps protect the organs

- Helps the body to eliminate toxins and wastes
- Aides in transportation of nutrients and oxygen
- Aides in digestion and metabolism
- Keeps your skin looking younger
- And to summarize some information you may like to know. Drinking enough water allows your kidney to function properly without help from the liver. This allows the liver to do one of its jobs, metabolizing fats. Taking in more water can also help flush out excess sodium which helps reduce water retention (bloating).

Chapter 6

Exercise

Chapter Highlights:

- Why aerobic exercise is important, and how to set your target heart rate (THR).

- Why weight training is necessary for success.

- What type of weight training will produce optimal results.

There are more articles about the benefits of both cardiovascular and weight-training exercise than you could ever imagine. New research continues to find further evidence that not only supports what we already know, it also points towards even further protection from degenerative diseases. Below are just some of the major benefits for anyone who has not read those articles:

- Improved Cardiovascular Function (allows the heart to supply more O_2 with less effort)
  - improves blood lipid profile (i.e., increases HDL [good] cholesterol, reduces LDL [bad] cholesterol)
  - decreases blood pressure
  - improves glucose metabolism
  - reduces likelihood of a cardiovascular event (heart attack, stroke, etc.)

- Reduced Risk of Osteoporosis
  - bone mineral loss is slowed, or in some cases bone density is increased (bone is living tissue and will adapt and strengthen with resistance training)

- Increased Muscle Hypertrophy and Muscle Endurance
  - helps to create muscle tone and give the body shape and definition
  - increased muscle mass raises the basal metabolic rate
  - can help improve performance, balance, and coordination
  - reduces chance of injury and improves recovery time from injury

- Improved Body Composition
  - muscle mass increases and body fat is reduced

- Improved Self-Esteem

- Increased Energy and Stamina

As you can see, exercise has some important benefits. However, no amount of exercise can make up for not fueling your body properly. Do not forget, your foundation begins with nutrition. Your body's engine is its metabolism. The combination of nutrition and exercise is your key to getting results. We want to rev up that engine to get a higher output of calories, and exercise is one of the best ways to accomplish this. The most common excuse for neglecting our health is the time factor. "I don't have enough time", is one of the worst ones out there. To put things in perspective, did you know that it only requires 2% of your time to follow the surgeon general's guidelines for exercise? You should also know that the more you exercise, the more energy you will have, and the less you exercise, the less energy you will have. It has been proven that fit people are more productive and efficient with their time. Think of exercise as a small time investment which will produce great returns by making you more efficient, productive, and may also add 10–15 years to your life. This should make up for the time you spend working out in the long run, so now who doesn't have time?

Aerobic Exercise
(Cardio)

While aerobics may be an extremely important piece of the fitness equation, to borrow a quote from Dr. Kenneth Cooper (the father of aerobic exercise), "Aerobics are merely the foundation for a good exercise program." There are still too many individuals out there who overemphasize aerobic exercise and miss out on the benefits of resistance training. The media have come around over the past

5 years or so and have begun to tout the importance of weight training. Unfortunately, not everyone has gotten the message. Have you ever known a fairly serious runner or an aerobics-class veteran who fits the following profile? They eat well, yet can't seem to tone up and get the look they desire. They are what I call "skinny fat" people. They are generally slim, but have very little muscle tone. The ones who don't eat well are a huskier version of the same flabby body. The reason this occurs is that muscle gives our body its form and shape. Without it there is not much under the skin but fat and bones. This becomes even more pronounced as we age and body parts begin to lose their battle with gravity. This is because once we reach our thirties, if we are not lifting weights, the body will begin to lose muscle at a rate of 0.5–1 pound per year. Our runner friend can run all he wants, but he can't run away from the effects of aging. The only way to escape the rounded shoulders, sagging chest, and that big saggy lump of fat on the back of the arms is to fight these effects with weight lifting. We will get into how to accomplish this when we finish the aerobics section.

By now you may be wondering whether or not aerobic exercise is all that important. Well, it is—but no more so than weight training or getting proper nutrition. It is one of the most important things for you to do if you want to be healthy, lean, and fit. It is, after all, exercise for your heart. The heart is the most important muscle you have. The health benefits, which we covered earlier in this chapter, are tremendous. The performance and appearance benefits are equally amazing. Since the focus of this book is how to get you lean and fit, we will now discuss the purpose of doing aerobic exercise to reach this goal. Aerobic exercise is defined as a continuous activity that elevates the heart rate to a given intensity for a minimum of 20 minutes. It is around the 20-minute mark that muscle glycogen stores diminish and your body begins to draw more energy from fat. This fat is released from the cells for your muscles to burn as fuel. There are a variety of activities that can qualify, but to keep things simple, walking, running, biking, elliptical training, and swimming are your most common modes. While you are performing these activities, you are burning calories. More importantly, you are burning fat. The key is to do it right. You need the appropriate frequency, intensity, and duration for your body.

The American College of Sports Medicine (ACSM) guidelines for general health and fitness are 3–5 days per week (frequency), and 20–60 minutes per day (duration). If your goal is weight loss, you will need to exercise aerobically for longer than 40 minutes per day or more than 5 days per week or both. Unfortunately, most Americans are not getting anywhere near this amount of aerobic exercise, let alone doing it optimally. If you want to achieve results, you need to have a program that will fit into your lifestyle. When I sit down with a client to design a program for them, I need to know what they have done in the past, what they are doing now, and whether or not it is working for them. This information will help me determine the best possible routine. There are several choices to make regarding your mode of exercise. If you want to keep the price low, buy some running shoes and walk or run outside. If you have knee or other joint problems, you need to reduce joint impact and would be better off on an elliptical trainer or a bike. On the other hand, if you enjoy running, but can't find the time to get out of the house because of the kids, you should purchase a treadmill. You need to think about which mode will be best for you before you start your routine. Once I have helped the client remove all barriers (excuses) for not getting a workout in, I will design a routine. If I have a client who is already doing 4 days of cardio per week for 40 minutes per session, I may push them to 5 days and 45–50 minutes. On the other hand, if I have a client who is currently doing nothing, anything would be an improvement. I may start them off at only 3 days and 20–30 minutes to see how their body responds and adjust accordingly.

Intensity is an extremely important factor in customizing your program. Training at the right intensity will ensure you maximize your benefits while still exercising safely. To truly know your appropriate intensity you need to have an exercise test performed in a clinical setting. Although this is recommended before starting an exercise program for those over 50 years of age or with known heart disease, it is not practical for everyone. Another way to find your training intensity or Target Heart Rate (THR) is to use a calculation called the Karvonen formula (see table below). Before doing this, one must know their resting heart rate (RHR). If you know how to check your pulse or have access to a heart rate monitor, you can make the calculations. Once you know your RHR, you can calculate a range for your THR. The THR range is calculated at 50% to 85% intensity for beginners through advanced exercisers whose goal is burning body fat. Anything above this intensity will put your body into an anaerobic state (without oxygen) and your body cannot burn fat without oxygen. When setting your intensity level it is always best to underestimate your fitness level and adjust intensity up as needed. This is much safer than pushing too hard and risking injury or cardiovascular incident.

Maximum HR	= 220 - Age	220 - 40 yrs.	= 180
HR reserve	= Maximum HR - RHR	180 - 70 bpm	= 110
Intensity	= HR reserve × 50 - 85%	110 × 0.7	= 77
THR	= Intensity + RHR	77 + 70	= 147 bpm

Note: If you are on any medications, such as beta blockers, that may affect your heart rate response to exercise, your THR will need to be adjusted.

While the Karvonen Formula is a great way to estimate your THR, it is only an estimation. It has a margin of error of up to 30 beats a minute. Obviously starting low and working your way up can become a trial and error process. What is most important is how you feel at a given intensity of work. There is a scale of intensity called the Borg Scale (see insert below) which helps you to determine your perceived level of work. Using both the THR and Borg Scale in combination is a better way to determine your appropriate intensity. You eventually want to work-out at a level where you are breathing heavier, but can still talk if necessary.

	Official	Commonsense	Where you should be
6		lying in bed	
7	very, very light		
8			
9	very light	walking to car	
10			
11	fairly light		beginners
12		brisk walk	
13	somewhat hard		
14		can talk, but not hold	intermediate
15	hard	a full conversation	
16			
17	very hard	sweating heavier	advanced
18			
19	very, very hard		very fit
20		can't speak, need rest	

The importance of appropriate intensity cannot be overstated. We need to make sure you are exercising at a high enough level to make it worth your time, but not so intense that you risk injury or cardiovascular incident. Remember, working out at a higher intensity allows you to burn more calories in less time, but this carries an additional risk if you are not properly conditioned. The following is an example of a client who was not maximizing their time:

Pam was a perfect example of someone who was doing 4 days of cardio each week, but not really getting much benefit from it. She did her walks in the morning with a friend, and they enjoyed each other's company. They also probably kept each other accountable to doing the workouts, which is very important. Unfortunately, her 45-minute walks were more of a social event than a workout. One of the first things I had her do was wear a heart rate monitor and see what her heart rate was during the walks. I then calculated her target heart rate using the Karvonen formula. As I suspected, she had not been achieving her target heart rate during her walks. I then took her through a workout at the appropriate intensity so she could feel the difference and I could make sure she was able to handle the intensity. This is an extremely important point. You can use the formula to figure out what your hear rate "should" be, but the most important thing is how you actually feel. You may need to adjust your target heart rate up or down a bit to achieve an intensity level that works for you. You should feel as if you are working hard enough to break a sweat, but you should still be able to speak fairly easily. If you are huffing and puffing, you may be pushing too hard.

The key to burning off fat is creating a gap between calories in and calories out. If we adjust your diet and you consume 250 fewer calories per day than your metabolic rate, we can create a weekly gap of 1,750 calories. If we then have you do cardio 5 days per week and you burn 350 calories per session, you now have another 1,750 gap. This adds up to a weekly gap of 3,500 calories, which would be a 1-pound fat loss per week.

In appendix III you will find four fitness categories. Match the appropriate category to your fitness level and do not overestimate your ability. Once you determine your fitness category, you can move through the progression of a 12-week program.

Weight Training

Weight training or resistance training, whatever you call it, involves moving a muscle against a force. This action results in the muscle tissue breaking down and rebuilding stronger. The muscle will continue to rebuild stronger as long as the stimulus placed on it is progressively increased (this is the progressive overload principle). The increased stimulus forces muscle, as well as bone, to adapt. One of the biggest mistakes beginners make is to learn one routine when they first start out and to continue with it indefinitely. When this occurs, the individual experiences some results in the beginning, but eventually plateaus. Many times these plateaus can last a very long time. The person keeps going to the gym and doing the same old routine without any further results. On the positive side, the exerciser is still benefiting their health to a degree, but this can become very frustrating and some people may eventually quit. Just as the mind can become bored doing the same thing over and over, the body can also become "bored" and eventually stops producing results. Our bodies are very efficient; without variety in your exercise routine, you will not stimulate the muscles enough to adapt and change.

The progressive overload does not only come from increasing the resistance. This may come as a relief to any of you who still hold the belief that weight training will make you "bulky." This myth will only become a reality if you fail to eat properly or fail to perform your cardio routine on a regular basis. You can achieve progressive overload by creating a variety of stimuli. Anything from changing your repetition and set ranges to changing your actual exercises will suffice. Changing your exercises means, for example, going from a bench press as your primary chest exercise to a dumbbell press or going from a dumbbell bicep curl to a cable curl. These seemingly minor changes will force your muscles to keep adapting and will keep you moving towards your goal.

Before we move on, some of the other myths that still exist about weight training need to be dispelled. If it's not the "big and bulky" myth, it's the belief that aerobic exercise is all one needs. This could not be further from the truth. A runner will become a better and more powerful runner if they train properly. And the "skinny fat person" becomes the "skinny fat person" by not doing resistance training. The effects of not training mentioned in the aerobics section were more short-term and appearance-oriented. If we fast-forward 30–40 years, the effects are far worse. Currently, 25% of men and 66% of women age 75 and up cannot lift an object heavier than 10 pounds (Framingham, Mass., Study of Physical

Disability Among the Aging). Think of how it would affect your quality of life if you could not lift your own groceries or grandchildren. Think of the burden you will become to your family or to the health care workers who need to move you out of bed because you are too heavy and weak to move on your own.

Those statistics are the main reason the American College of Sports Medicine (ACSM) added weight training to their list of recommend exercises for overall fitness. The ACSM recommends a minimum training stimulus of one set of 8–12 repetitions for 8–10 muscle groups 2 days per week. This is the minimum. Nearly every study ever published has shown 3 sets to be more effective than 1 set. You may have tried or heard about single-set routines that can save you time. They claim you can get in one or two workouts per week in just 20–30 minutes apiece. The movements are super-slow and very controlled. This type of workout will allow you to feel a good muscle "burn". However, it is best suited for those rehabilitating from an injury or teaching a newcomer proper form—results will be limited. Another time saving program that is extremely popular has become one of the nation's fastest-growing chains. You see them in just about every shopping plaza these days, but don't let this women's-only program throw you a curve ball. While this program is a great way to get started for someone who does not have much exercise experience, that is about all it will do for you. Those who stick with it will eventually plateau. You can only do so much in a ½ hour. When part of this time is dedicated to cardio circuit training it is not enough time to progress a full-body workout.

In defense of the single set advocates, I will admit that you can achieve some results on those types of programs. In fact studies have shown that just about <u>any</u> program will bring about <u>initial</u> results in an untrained body. If you are short on time, something is always better than nothing. However, the question I have for you is, how fast do you want your results, and how far do you want to take them? Nobody would buy a car that they knew would only last for 5000 miles and nobody should choose a program that will give them limited results. Remember, this program is designed to give you optimal long term results.

We have already covered the fact that multiple sets are superior to single sets. To be more specific, studies also show that beginners will respond best to a resistance of 60% of their maximum strength for a given exercise if they train their body parts 3 days per week. This usually equates to a range of 15–25 repetitions. After that you must increase your intensity. More advanced exercisers will need to train at around 80% of their maximum strength, or 8–12 repetitions. This is difficult to do with the equipment used at most circuit-training facilities, and especially at the pace of a circuit-training workout. The exercise recommendations also call for only 2 days per week for each body part because at this higher intensity the body requires more recovery time between sets as well as between workouts.

Note: You should never train the same muscle groups 2 days in a row, when you lift weights, you actually break down the muscle fibers and they need about 48 hours to repair themselves.

There are many variables to designing an exercise routine that will provide the results you are looking for. Depending on your training goals, you should typically change some aspect of your routine about every four to six weeks. When designing an exercise program you first must decide on what your goal is and what your time frame should be to meet this goal. This program will last for 12-weeks, divided up into four 3-week sections. Each section is specific to a certain type of development and not everyone will move through it the same. If someone is deconditioned they may need more work on building a foundation and will need to spend more time in the first phase before moving on to the next. On the other hand if you are fairly well conditioned from past training and injury-free you can probably move through the first phase in only 2 weeks. Everyone has different genetics and therefore responds differently to a particular type of program. This program has been designed to help you become lean and fit. Specific stages offer alternative choices to help you customize the plan to your body and keep moving towards your specific goal.

As you can see, it takes a bit more to design a routine that will deliver the results you are looking for. However, it is well worth the effort and far better than just going to the gym and going through the motions. Appendix IV & V contain the actual exercises and routines for each stage. These will give you a more detailed look at how to create the right program for your 12-week program.

Afterword

I hope the information I have provided will allow you to paint a clear picture of how you will create the new you. You should picture this person in your mind. Think about what you will be able to do, be able to wear, and how you will feel. Think about this person daily, because what we focus on, we tend to create. Whether you believe you can or you believe you can't, either way you are right. If you have doubts about whether this plan, or anything you do, is really going to work, these doubts will become a self-fulfilling prophecy. These doubts mean you are not ready or you are still holding on to a limiting belief ("I can't lose weight, I have bad genetics" or "Weight loss is difficult for me, I'm doomed for failure"). Such beliefs will cause you to consciously or unconsciously sabotage your program. Ask yourself the following questions:

- Do you believe that eating 4–6 balanced meals per day will help you become leaner?
- Do you believe doing cardio 3–6 days per week for 40–60 minutes in your target heart rate zone will help you to burn body fat?
- Do you believe that a periodized weight training plan will help you gain muscle tissue, which will in turn give your body more tone and a higher metabolism?

If this all makes sense to you, then you are ready to start your program.

If this does not make sense to you, it's okay— not everyone is at a point in their life where they can take on a challenge like this. You do not want to just try this program; you need to fully experience it, because no program will work if you are not prepared to complete it. I have seen clients who were not ready to commit to their program. They said they were, but they were not being honest with themselves. They made an attempt, but did not really have the intent to succeed. It was much easier to blame some unforeseen circumstances on why they could not do it. If you really do make the attempt, you will find out whether or not you can do it.

"I'll try it" is a self-protection mechanism that prevents you from ever facing confirmation of failure. If you are afraid of failure, you will probably never taste success. If you happen to fall into this category, you may want to take some time to get organized and prepared, so that when you do start the program you can do it successfully.

Once you reach the point of truly being ready, and have selected your goals, it's time to commit to them. This is a very powerful word. If you look in the dictionary, you'll see the definitions "to entrust or to pledge to oneself," "to bind," "to perform," and "to do." Commit and you will give yourself the chance to truly experience your potential and get the results you desire. Think about how long it took you to get to where you are. It will also take some time to reach your goal, although not nearly as long. Select a qualified trainer, if necessary, and plan on spending some time with that person. It may take time to learn all the proper techniques. Sometimes people think they can make it on their own before they are really ready. A trainer can help monitor your progress, hold you accountable, and prevent you from falling into some of the same old habits. This can be an invaluable service when it comes to ensuring your success as well as your safety. As you do begin to see results, you should reward yourself for your accomplishments. When you drop a few sizes, get a new outfit. If you put in a few good weeks, schedule a massage for those muscles you have been working. Treat yourself in ways that will improve your health and appearance, because it will do you no good to indulge in things that will reduce the benefits you have worked for. Enjoy the program, enjoy the results, treat yourself well, and tell others to get on THE PROGRAM.

Appendix I

Food Choice List

To begin this program you must first take a look at the list of foods below, pick the ones you like and use them to create a balanced meal, actually 4–6 balanced meals. One thing I always explain to my clients with this list is that there are plenty of great choices on the list, but this does not mean this is all that you can ever eat. If you feel the need to eat something that is not on the list, whether it is "bad" or not, do not "deprive" yourself of it. Depriving oneself of a "forbidden food" will only increase temptation. Just recognize what you are eating and think about whether you really want it or not. Having a small controlled amount is better than binging on a large amount. For example, if you have a weakness for ice-cream, instead of keeping ice cream in your freezer go out and get a small cone once in awhile.

Poultry	Meat	Cereals	Vegetables
Chicken	Buffalo	Corn Flakes	Artichoke
Turkey	Venison	Cheerios™	Asparagus
Egg Whites		Cream of Wheat™	Bean Sprouts
Ostrich	**Starch**	Fiber One™	Beets
	Barley	Great Grains (Post™)	Broccoli
Fish	Beans	Kashi GoLean™	Brussel Sprouts
Tuna	Bread (oat bran/rye)	Kashi Puffed™	Carrots
Alaskan Salmon	Corn	Oatmeal	Cauliflower
Mahi Mahi	Peas	Shredded Wheat™	Cucumber
Tilapia	Potato (sweet)	Uncle Sam's™	Mushrooms
Flounder	Quinoa		Salad Greens
Cod	Rice (Brown/Wild)		Soybeans
Shrimp	Wheat Pasta		Spinach
White Fish	Yam		Tomato
			Zucchini

Fruits
Apple
Banana
Blackberries
Cantaloupe
Cherries
Grapefruit
Grapes
Kiwi
Mango
Melon
Nectarine
Orange
Peach
Pear
Pineapple

Plums
Raisins
Strawberries
Tangerines
Watermelon

Nuts/Grains/Fats
Almonds
Cashews
Walnuts
Waffles
Almond Butter
Peanut Butter
Olive oil & Vinegar
Flaxseed/oil

Supplements
Whey Protein
IronTek Protein™
LeanBody Shakes™
Myo-plex Shakes™
Balance Bar Gold™
Gourmet Bar™
Myo-plex Lite™
Parillo Bar™
Organic Bar
Pure Protein™
Zone Bar™

Other
Cottage Cheese
1% or Skim Milk
Yogurt (low-fat)
Soy Milk

Appendix II

Meal Planner

One thing we need to discuss in detail is how to design and balance these meals once you know what your caloric intake should be. For example, Tammy from the nutrition chapter requires 1400 calories per day to lose 1 pound per week. We can now figure this out on a per meal and per day basis. If Tammy's schedule only allows for 5 meals per day, we can divide 1400 by 5 and get 280 calories per meal. Based on the formula using 1–1.5 grams per pound of lean body weight, Tammy should eat 80–120 grams of protein per day. If she decides to eat 100 grams of protein, this would equate to 400 calories from protein per day or 20 grams and 80 calories per meal. From here we can also divide 400 calories by 1400 and see that 28.5% of total intake is from protein. Summary below:

1400 calories/5 meals = 280 calories per meal
100 grams of protein/5 meals = 20 grams per meal
100 grams protein X 4 calories per gram = 400 calories
400 calories/1400 calories = 28.5% of calories from protein.

Recommended ranges for all phases of this program:	
Protein	- 25–35%
Fats	- 15–30%
Carbs	- 40–60%

Note: These do not exactly follow the USDA dietary guidelines which recommend a lower protein intake along with a slightly higher fat and carbohydrate intake.

Next we can figure her fat intake; 15–30% of caloric intake is usually a good range for a fat loss program. If we use 25% of total calories for Tammy, or 25% of

1400, we get 350 calories. Divide this by 9 calories per gram and we get about 39 grams of fat per day.

Fat Reference Chart:	(percentage of intake)			
	30%	20%	10%	
1500 calorie intake =	50g	33g	16g	(g per/day)
2000 calorie intake =	66g	44g	22g	

Carbohydrates will then make up the other 46.5% of caloric intake which is 650 calories or 162.5 grams.

Note: I have provided this information so that you can better understand this process; however, you really do not need to do all of this. As long as you figure your protein intake and you eat balanced meals such as the ones in the menu guidelines, you will fall into the range of 15–30% for fats, 25–35% for proteins, and 40–60% for carbohydrates.

If you are on the Jump Start Plan you will be towards the higher end of the range on the protein and fats, and lower on the carbs. As you move through the phases your % of carb intake should increase accordingly. Since the Jump Start plan is going to provide less energy, it would best suit beginners whose overall exercise intensity will not be all that high in the beginning. More experienced exercisers who decide to begin at higher training intensities may want to start with the Steady Pace plan. You should remain on this plan until you achieve your goal weight/fat loss goal. If at the end of the 12 week program you are looking for additional fat loss you could also try cycling in the Jump Start plan. This can be done 2–3 days per week by eating Steady Pace Mon, Wed, Fri, and Sat. and then eating Jump Start Tue, Thurs, and Sun.

Although the Steady Pace already provides an ample amount of carbohydrates for most people, and could even be considered a maintenance phase for some individuals, the Maintenance Phase is for those who have progressed to a high activity level. Those who would like to add more muscle mass or workout more intensely will need the additional carbohydrates to provide the extra calories and energy needed.

The progression through each phase will take you to your goal and help you maintain that achievement. As you move through each phase you will get a better sense of what the appropriate amount of food for your body is and you will not need to keep measuring your portion sizes, although I highly recommend this in the beginning.

For any of you who would like to keep track of food intake with some accuracy, but without all the detail, the American Dietetic Association & American Diabetes Association created a Food Values Chart. This chart, or system, breaks all foods down into 6 basic categories and several subcategories allowing you to quickly determine the approximate nutritional value of each meal.

Meat: (1oz serving of lean, medium, and high fat)
  <u>Lean</u> = 55 calories, 7 grams protein, 3 grams fat; ex. (chicken, turkey, buffalo, most fish)
  <u>Med.</u> = 75 calories, 7 grams protein, 5 grams fat; ex. (beef, pork, salmon, low fat cheese)
  <u>High</u> = 100 calories; (not recommended)

Milk: (1cup) <u>Skim</u> = 90 calories, 12 grams carbohydrate, 8 grams protein
     <u>Low</u> = 120 calories, 12 grams carbohydrate, 8 grams protein, 5 grams fat
    <u>Whole</u> = 150 calories (not recommended)

Starch: (1 slice bread) = 80 calories, 15 grams carbohydrate, 3 grams protein

Fat: (1 teaspoon oil) = 45 calories, 5 grams fat

Fruit: (1 medium piece) = 60 calories, 15 grams carbohydrate

Vegetable: (1 cup raw) = 25 calories, 5 grams carbohydrate, 2 grams protein

Example: How many calories is this lunch, 4oz turkey on 2 slices of rye bread, with 2 cups salad and 2 teaspoons olive oil and vinegar?

4oz lean meat, 4 x 55 = 220 calories 2 cups vegetable, 2 x 25 = 50 calories
2 slices bread, 2 x 80 = 160 calories 2 teaspoons fat, 2 x 45 = 90 calories
              TOTAL = 520 calories

You can also use this information to figure out approximately how many grams of protein, carbs and fat you are eating.

Jump Start Meals

Note on all meals and recipes: The following meals are for one person serving sizes. If you are going to cook for more, increase proportions accordingly. The recipes (when provided are kept very simple as I am not the greatest of chefs. If you would like to "spice" any of these up with your on special touch do so without reducing the health value of the meal. I.e. Avoid the obvious, deep frying, heavy (high fat) sauces, mayonnaise...Do feel free to use mustard, horseradish, health cooking oils (olive, soybean,...) and your spice rack to flavor your foods.

Breakfast:

Eggs and fruit: Make a three egg scramble or omelet using 3 egg whites and 1 yolk. Mix in some veggies (tomatoes, onions, broccoli...) for additional nutrients and some low fat cheese if you like. Have a piece of fruit as well.

Cottage cheese & fruit: Mix ½ to 1 cup of low fat cottage cheese with your favorite fruit.

Lower Carb Smoothie: 4–5 strawberries blended with 1 cup of milk (skim, soy, or rice), 1 scoop of protein powder and a few ice cubes.

Snacks:

Tuna Mix: Tuna (3–6 oz) with diced tomatoes (1/2 cup) and balsamic vinaigrette (1 tbsp).

Cottage Cheese Mix: Low fat cottage cheese (½–1 cup) with cashews (1 tbsp).

Fruit & Nut Combo: Apple with peanut butter (1 tbsp) or some mixed nuts.

Buffalo Jerky (2–3 oz) and some mixed nuts (1–2 tbsp).

Lunch & Dinner: Rule of thumb (4–6 oz of meat with 2 cups of vegetables)
Fish, chicken, or steak (4–6 oz) with vegetables (2 cups) and a salad (2 cups).

Chicken tenders over bed of salad greens.

Chicken and shrimp Kabobs with peppers, onions, and tomatoes.

Chicken or steak and vegetable (onions, peppers, broccoli...) stir fry (no rice).

Steady Pace Meals

<u>Breakfast Meals:</u>
Oatmeal (½ cup) with blueberries (¼ cup), and egg whites (3)

Egg Sandwich: bread (2 slices), eggs (2 whites, 1 yolk) and fruit.

Dippy Eggs: Toast (1 slice), eggs over easy (3 whites, 1 yolk), and fruit.

Egg Scramble Special: In a frying pan (use cooking spray) cook diced potatoes and onions (1 cup), add in beaten eggs (3 whites, 1 yolk) and stir until cooked evenly. For added flavor add some low fat turkey sausage and/or peppers to the mix. Have one piece of fruit on the side.

<u>Smoothies:</u> Get your blender out.
Lower carb/calorie: 6–8 oz skim milk, 4–5 strawberries, 1 scoop protein powder.

6–8 oz skim milk, 1 cup frozen mixed berries, 1 scoop protein powder.

Mid-Calorie: 6oz yogurt, 3 strawberries, ¼ cup pineapple, small banana, 3 ice cubes, and 1 scoop protein powder.

6–8 oz skim milk, 4 strawberries, small banana, 1 scoop protein powder.

High-Calorie   6–8 oz milk, banana, 1 tablespoon peanut butter, 1–2 scoops protein powder.

<u>Snacks:</u>
Cottage Cheese Mix: Low fat cottage cheese (½ cup) with kashi cereal (½ cup) and berries.

2 Rice cakes with 2 tablespoons peanut butter.

Meal replacement bar or shake.

<u>Lunch:</u>
Fish or meat (4–6 oz) over rice (½ cup) or with baked potato and vegetables (1–2 cups)

Chicken or turkey (4–6 oz) sandwich with mustard and vegetables (1 cup) on side.

Turkey or Buffalo (4–6 oz) Burger and a salad (2 cups).

Chicken tenders (4–6 oz) over salad greens (2 cups) with a baked sweet potato.

Chicken (4–6 oz) and vegetable stir fry over rice (½ cup)

Dinner:

Fish, chicken, or steak with vegetables and a salad.

Chicken tenders over bed of salad greens.

Chicken and shrimp Kabobs with peppers, onions, and tomatoes.

Chicken or steak and vegetable stir fry (no rice)

Maintenance Phase

This phase is for when you have achieved the results you were looking for (weight/fat loss) and you are now looking to maintain those results long term. Use all of the already described meals in whatever combination you like best. Add whatever similar types of meals or recipes you know of; just make sure they follow the rules of being balanced. You should now use the lunches from steady pace plan as your dinner meals. This means you can also add complex carbs like rice and sweet potatoes or yams to your dinner meals. One particular favorite of mine is a baked sweet potato with cinnamon and butter. Feel free to mix it up. If you want to have a breakfast meal like the egg scramble special for dinner on occasion, go right ahead. As long as you continue to eat healthy nutritious foods (avoid going back to your old habits) you should have no problem maintaining your results.

Appendix III

Aerobic Exercise

In order to categorize your fitness level, read through the following selections and place yourself in the appropriate category.

Out of Shape (OOS):
Have not performed aerobic exercise >1 day per week in past 1 or more years.
Become out of breath quickly upon mild—moderate exertion
(Get doctors clearance before beginning)

Average American (AA):
Have not worked out regularly in past 3–6 months
Fatigue quickly with moderate exertion
(May also need doctors clearance before beginning)

Better than Average (BTA):
Work out 1–3 days per week for past 3–6 months
Can last for 20–40 minutes for cardio session

Healthy (H):
Regularly work out 3–5 days/week for past year or more
Have good stamina, just need a better routine

Whichever category you fit into, follow the F.I.T. (frequency, intensity, time) principle described in each section. You should also perform your routine when you wake up first thing in the morning before you have breakfast. There are two major reasons to do this. Several studies have shown that your body has less glycogen stores available after fasting all night. This allows your body to access its fat stores more quickly. Second, when you do this before anything else, it not only energizes you for your day, it also does not allow you to make an excuse for why you could not fit it into your schedule later on. Things are always going to "come up" in your life, creating this morning ritual will prevent these things from becoming a barrier to your success. Make it a habit to get up early enough so you can make this work and if that means going to bed a little earlier, than so be it.

Week 1–2 (OOS and AA): (remember to warm up thoroughly before going into your zone)
Frequency—3–4 days per week, preferably on days off from weight training.

Intensity—Using the Karvonen formula set your THR to 40–60% of max, Judge how you feel at this intensity and adjust as necessary. At the proper intensity you should still be able to talk, but not easily carry on a full conversation.

Time—Aim for 30–40 minutes. If you are deconditioned and do not have the endurance or just do not have the time, break up your routine into a morning and evening split, 15–20 minutes each. Remember, something is always better than nothing and you will eventually increase your duration.

Week 3–4 (OOS, AA, start point for BTA):
Gradually progress your workouts, don't forget your warm up.
Frequency—4–6 days

Intensity—If you felt you started too easy, you can move up to 60–70% of max.

Time—40–60 minutes (you can still split if necessary)

Week 5–8 (OOS, AA, BTA, start point for H):
Interval training.
Frequency—4 days (+2 days of week 3–4 routine if you have more than 20 lbs to lose or your body is responding slowly.)

Intensity—Use 75–85% for your high interval, and 55–65% for your low interval

Time—Perform a 5 minute warm-up, followed by a 2 minute high interval and a 3 minute low interval. Repeat the interval cycle 4–5 times for a total exercise time of 30–35 minutes.

Example: 5 minute warm-up (HR 130)
                 2 minutes high (HR 160)
                 3 minutes low (HR 120)
                 2 minutes high (HR 160)
                 3 minutes low (HR 120)
                 5–6 of each, your last low interval will be your cool-down.

Week 9–12 OOS and AA):

Continue with same routine. If you need to increase intensity, you can reduce the recovery time to 2 minutes and/or add a sixth or seventh high interval.

Week 9–12 (BTA and H):

Continue with similar routine, but switch high interval to 3 minutes and low to 2 minutes.

There are several ways to optimize your workouts for the best possible results:
- more = better (to a point): If one is already exercising and has a fitness base they should be able to max out their frequency at 6 days per week. The body requires some rest and you probably should not perform cardio every single day.

- getting the right intensity: The area of intensity is a bit more complex. A beginner should start out with long low-moderate intensity cardio workouts to maximize fat burning. A more advanced exerciser will benefit more from the interval sessions provided. These higher intensity sessions allow you to get the higher calorie burn during the high intensity portion and the higher percentage fat burn during the low intensity portion. Beginners should not attempt these types of workouts until they build up their fitness base.

- do your cardio when you are in a lower glycogen state; we already covered one time when this occurs (in the morning). The other is after your weight training workout. Weight training is an anaerobic exercise which will only burn blood sugars (from glycogen stores) leaving you in a lower glycogen state for your cardio workout and better able to tap into your fat stores. *Note: you should not do your cardio before weight training because you will burn your glycogen stores up and not have as much energy left over for your weight workout.*

Special Note on interval training: Interval workouts are a great way to get a higher overall calorie burn in a shorter period of time. There are many advantages to performing higher intensity workouts. Not only are your workouts shorter, but you actually have a greater improvement in overall cardiovascular capacity. These types of workouts also stimulate certain hormones in your body to create a greater overall effect. One such hormone is HGH or Human Growth Hormone. HGH is known as the anti-aging hormone and is sometimes injected by those who desire it's fat cutting, muscle toning, and rejuvenating properties. Although there is a decline in HGH secretion as we age, high intensity anaerobic exercise such as sprints and weight training can naturally increase our bodies own production of HGH. The cardio workouts I have provided are not considered high intensity anaerobic workouts. They are low to moderately high intensity aerobic workouts and are a necessary stepping stone to prepare you for higher intensity workouts. Many of you will feel that they are already fairly high intensity routines and will not need to look any further. For those who do wish to progress beyond what I have provided you must know that as the intensity increases, so does the risk. It could be the risk of a skeletal or muscular injury or possibly a heart attack. You should check with your doctor and seek out the advice of a conditioning coach or trainer before taking on this type of activity.

Appendix IV

12 Week Resistance Routine

Before you begin your weight training program you should consult a doctor about any injuries or medical conditions that may limit your ability to perform a particular exercise. You should also use the fitness categories below to place yourself in the appropriate starting point.

Out of Shape (OOS):
Have not performed weight lifting exercises at all in the past 1 or more years. Have very little or no experience using free weights or weights in general.

Those who fall into this category probably do not have a high level of muscular coordination. You will feel more comfortable and probably be safer using weight machines before moving on to free weights. Machines are great at isolating particular muscle groups, thus allowing the beginner to feel the working muscle. You can then transition to using free weights which offer greater range of motion, use of stabilizing muscle groups and movements that translate into real life activities. You should start with **Phase Ia**.

Average American (AA):
Have not worked out regularly in past 3–6 months
Cannot pass the following test: (exercises are listed in appendix V)

Upper Body—regular Pushups (men), Knee Pushups (women) for at least 10 reps.
Core—Perform 20 continuous basic crunches with good form.
Lower Body—Perform Ball Squats for at least 20 reps.

If you cannot pass this test, start with **Phase Ia,** if you barely passed **Ib**.

Better than Average (BTA):
>   Work out 1–3 days per week for past 3–6 months
>   You probably passed the test quite easily because you have a decent fitness base.
>   You can start with either **Phase Ib** or **Ic.**

Healthy (H):
>   Regularly work out 3–5 days/week for past year or more.
>   You probably have a good fitness base and are looking to fine tune your workout or get more defined than you currently are. If Phase I is similar to your current program, you may want to begin with **Phase II,** if not **Ic** is a good starting place.

Now we are ready to begin. If you have not purchased or created a journal to log your activities, I must remind you that tracking your workouts is very helpful in the process of progressing your workouts properly.

PHASE I: Adaptation (1–4 Weeks)

The purpose of this phase is to build a foundation of muscle strength and endurance as well as to work on technique and flexibility. To build up your muscle endurance we will be lifting with lighter weights and higher repetition counts. This will better prepare your muscles, ligaments, and tendons for the later phases. We will also add some circuit training and cardio intervals to boost your overall calorie burn during the workout and improve your overall conditioning. Although there will be some significant strength gains during this period, the focus is on proper form and technique. Besides form, two important techniques for you to learn are proper breathing and the mind-muscle connection. The correct way to breathe when you are lifting weights is to exhale with effort. When you are lifting a weight and it begins to get difficult, you should exhale. It is important to not hold one's breath while lifting. This creates what is called the Valsalva maneuver and can cause dangerous increases in your blood pressure. You do not have to make a huge effort or lots of noise when you breathe out, just breathe naturally until you form your own technique. The second technique you must learn is the mind-muscle connection. Basically this is about focusing on and visualizing the working muscle contractions. You must force them to work harder than they need to. Many times beginners just go through the motions. If you learn this technique you will get much more out of your workouts. The biceps curl is the easiest way to describe this process. If you have ever flexed your biceps when someone asked you to "make a muscle", you know how to consciously contract a muscle without resistance. The idea behind the mind-muscle connection is to consciously squeeze the working muscles harder than they need to, while lifting a weight. This is a technique that will come easy with some exercises and be very difficult with others, do not get discouraged, just keep practicing or ask for help from a fitness professional.

Two more important parts of this and every phase is to warm up for a few minutes before you begin your routine, and to increase flexibility. To make your workouts more efficient you should stretch the muscles worked between sets of those exercises. For example if you are doing leg extensions, stretch your quadriceps. Each stretch should be held for 15–30 seconds and repeated at least once. There is a guide to stretching in appendix V.

Type of Routine	- *Full Body with Circuit Training and/or Cardio Intervals
Frequency	- 2 to 3 days per week (2 x/week for beginners until week 3)
Intensity	- 60 % of max or 15–20 reps
Volume	- 2 to 3 sets per exercise, 1–2 exercises per muscle group
Rest Time	- 30–45 seconds between sets, use this time to stretch
Progression	- Select a weight you can perform 45–60 reps within three sets when you exceed 60 reps, increase to a heavier weight.

Exercise Routine for Phase Ia: (OOS and AA. You should remain in this phase for 1–2 weeks before moving on to Ib)

Chest:	Bench/Chest Press
Legs:	Leg Extension
Back:	Lat Pull down
Legs:	Ball Squat
Shoulders:	Lateral Raise
Triceps:	Triceps Pushdown
Biceps:	Dumbbell Curl
Core:	Basic Crunches

Note: If you cannot perform any of the exercises due to injury or equipment limitations, just select an alternative from the **exercise list section**. The overall plan is to perform 1–2 exercises per muscle group and complete 2–3 sets of each exercise (chest press), before moving on to the second (leg ext.).

Exercise Routine for Phase Ib: (Start point for BTA, AA. Week 2 or 3 for OOS, AA. Remain in this phase for 1–2 weeks, before moving on to Ic.)

Chest:	Bench/Chest Press
Legs:	Leg Extension
Back:	Lat Pull down
Legs:	Ball Squat
Shoulders:	Lateral Raise
Triceps:	Triceps Pushdown
Biceps:	Dumbbell Curl
Core:	Modified Crunch

Note: Pair off (super set) the two exercises, resting only after the second one in each group.

Exercise Routine for Phase Ic: (Start point for BTA,H. All should remain in this phase for 2 weeks before moving on to phase II)

Chest:	Bench/Chest Press
Legs:	Leg Extension
Cardio:	2 minute interval
Back:	Lat Pull down
Legs:	Ball Squat
Cardio:	2 minute interval
Shoulders:	Lateral Raise
Triceps:	Triceps Pushdown
Cardio:	2 minute interval
Biceps:	Dumbbell Curl
Core:	Ball Crunch

Note: Add the cardio interval as you become better conditioned, Use 60–70% THR.

PHASE II: Endurance/Hypertrophy (3–4 weeks)

While continuing to improve muscle endurance you will build more strength and muscle mass in this phase. This stage involves more advanced exercises and weight increases. You will begin to incorporate more free weight exercises (if you have not already) as your muscle coordination has improved. There will be no more circuit training or cardio intervals here. Your muscles will need all available oxygen for lifting the weights at this higher intensity. This phase will begin to really sculpt your body.

Type of Routine	- 2 day split routine (half one day, half the next)
Frequency	- 3 days per week (week 1—A, B, A week 2—B, A, B)
Intensity	- 60–70 % of max or 10–15 reps
Volume	- 3 sets per exercise, 2–4 exercises per muscle group.
Rest Time	- 45–60 seconds between sets, use this time to stretch
Progression	- Select a weight you can perform 30–45 reps within three sets when you exceed 45 reps, increase to the next weight.

Exercise routine for Phase II:

Workout A		Workout B	
Chest:	Incline Press	Back:	Lat Pull Down
	Dumbbell Fly		Seated Row
Shoulders:	Overhead Press	Biceps:	Dumbbell Curl
	Lateral Raise		Reverse Curl
Triceps:	Rope Pull downs	Legs:	Leg Extension
	Kickbacks		Leg Press
			Leg Curl

Phase III: Hypertrophy (2–4 weeks)

By now some muscles may begin to show through as you have lost enough body fat to reveal what you are sculpting. Depending on genetics and your overall goal, you may want to stay in this phase for a longer period of time while others may want to make it brief. For the latter, do not skip this phase, as it is very important in your development. Muscles do not appear over night, if you feel you are "overdeveloping" you can always lighten your weights and perform more reps. We are going to increase the volume of work here as well as apply the pyramid method. This is when you start with a lighter weight with your first set and gradually increase it in the following sets. As the weights get heavier the reps decrease.

Type of Routine	- 2 day split routine (2 different workouts)
Frequency	- 4 days per week (week 1—A1, B1, A2, B2)
Intensity	- 70–90 % of max or 6–12 reps
Volume	- 3–4 sets per exercise, 2–4 exercises per muscle group.
Rest Time	- 60–90 seconds between sets, use this time to stretch
Progression	- Pyramid your weights. Example; set 1 = 10lb x 12 reps Set 2, 12lb x 10 reps, set 3 15lb x 8 reps

Exercise routine for Phase III:

Workout A1

Chest	Bench Press
	Incline Dumbbell Press
Shoulders	Shoulder Press
	Shrugs
Triceps	Triceps Push Downs
	Dips

Workout B1

Back	Lat Pull Down
	Seated Row (narrow grip)
Biceps	EZ Curl
	Hammer Curl
Legs	Squats
	Leg Press

Workout A2

Chest	Dumbbell Fly
	Pushups
Shoulders	Lateral Raise
	Front Raise
Triceps	Skull Crushers
	Kickbacks

Workout B2

Back	Seated Row (wide grip)
	Reverse Fly
Biceps	Reverse EZ Curl
	Preacher Curl
Legs	Leg Extension
	Lunges
	Leg Curls

Phase IV: Finishing Phase (2–4 weeks)

Depending on your goal and your progress this will vary. If you would like to add more muscle mass 8–12 reps should be your goal. If you are looking to build more strength 6–8 reps, and if you want to maintain what you have achieved and just get leaner, increase reps to 20–30. We are going to a three day split here. This means shorter workouts that are focused on only 2 body parts.

Type of Routine	- 3 day split routine
Frequency	- 3–4 days per week (week 1—A, B, C, A…)
Intensity	- 50–90 % of max or 6–20 reps
Volume	- 3–4 sets per exercise, 2–4 exercises per muscle group.
Rest Time	- 45–90 seconds between sets, use this time to stretch
Progression	- continue with pyramids, increase weights as you exceed your rep ranges.

Exercise routine for Phase IV:

Workout A
Chest — Dumbbell Press / Incline Fly / Pushups

Triceps — Triceps Push Down / Skull Crushers / Kickbacks

Workout B
Back — Lat Pull down / Seated Row / Reverse Fly

Biceps — EZ Curl / Reverse EZ Curl / Preacher Curl

Workout C
Shoulders — Shoulder Press / Shrugs / Lateral Raise

Legs — Leg Extension / Squats / Lunges / Leg Curl

Beyond the 12 week program:

This program is really about making a life long change. Whether or not you still have further weight to lose after 12 weeks you should keep following the program. As you learned in the earlier chapters you should not have lost much more than 25 pounds of body fat during this process. If you do still have more to lose I would suggest you restart the program by following the nutrition suggestions at the end of appendix II and restart the exercise plan beginning at a higher intensity level. For cardio and weights try cycling through the last two phases and create your own 6 week program. For those of you who did reach their goal that does not mean you are finished. You now have the privilege of maintaining your achievement. You may want to challenge yourself with an occasional 3 or 6 week program.

This book has hopefully provided you with a toolbox full of exercises from which you can select the right ones to do the job. Try some that you may not have during the first program and find what works best for you. Beyond that, there are more ways to step up your training intensity and continue your progress. A few of the techniques you could employ include super sets, drop sets, and pre-fatigue sets. Supers sets are when you pair off 2 exercises of opposing muscle groups such as going from triceps right into bicep curls. This allows you to speed through a workout at a fast pace. Drop sets are when you force out additional reps with a lighter weight. For example if you are doing leg extensions and you do 12 reps at 100 pounds, immediately drop 30% to 70 pounds and get another 6–8 reps. You could even do a double drop to 50 pounds for an extra burn. Pre-fatiguing a muscle involves doing an isolation exercise before a compound exercise. Such as leg extensions right into leg presses. To learn more about these techniques as well as more advanced exercises I suggest you check out what some refer to as the "bible of weight training". Arnold Schwarzenegger wrote a book about all aspects of weight training. It is a very thorough book (approximately 800 pages) and is an excellent resource if you are looking for more information on advancing your training.

Appendix V

Exercise List

General form recommendations:
Good posture is a must with performing weight training exercises. Without it, injuries can occur. Remember these rules and you will be covered for most exercises.

1. Keep the head and neck in a neutral position unless specifically instructed otherwise.
2. The chest up, shoulders back "military form" position should be maintained with nearly every exercise.
3. Never "lock out" the joints. There are almost no situations in which you should completely straighten your elbows or knees. You should keep constant tension on the muscles for a better and safer workout.
4. Move through the full range of motion in a reasonably slow and controlled manor.
5. Whenever possible use a workout partner or trainer as a spotter.

(Pictures for most exercises listed below can be found on the following pages.)

	Machines	Free Weights	No/minimal Equipment
Chest	Chest press	Dumbbell Press	Pushups
	Smith Press (F, I, D)	*(F, I, D)	(wall, Knees, Ball)
	Pec Deck	Dumbbell Fly	
		Bench Press	* F, I, D = flat, incline, decline
Back	Lat Pull Down	1-Arm Row	Pull ups/Chin ups
	(wide or reverse grip)	Bent Over Row	
	Seated Row	Reverse Fly	
	Reverse Pec Deck		
Legs	Leg Press	Squats/Smith	Ball/Chair Squats
	Leg Extension	Lunges	Ball Leg Curl
	Leg Curls		Calves (heel raises)
Shoulders	Machine Press	Shoulder Press	Cord Lateral Raise
	Smith Shrugs	Lateral Raise	
		Shrugs	
Triceps	Cable Pushdown	Skull crushers	Dips
	(rope or bar)	Kickbacks	
	Cable Skull crushers		
Biceps	Cable Curl	Straight bar curl	Cord Curls
	Preacher machine	EZ curl or reverse curls	
		Db curl	
Abdominals	Crunch Machine	Slant board	Crunch
	Rope Crunch	Reverse crunch	V-up
			Ball
			Oblique

Barbell Bench Press & Smith Machine Press

- hand position should be approximately shoulder width
- the bar should line up with the midline of your chest
- place feet up on bench to reduce lower back arching
- lower bar until it is approximately 0–2 inches from chest
- press back up through a full range of motion until arms are nearly straight

*For those of you who are new to weight lifting the smith machine in the bottom picture works on a fixed path and is easier to learn with.

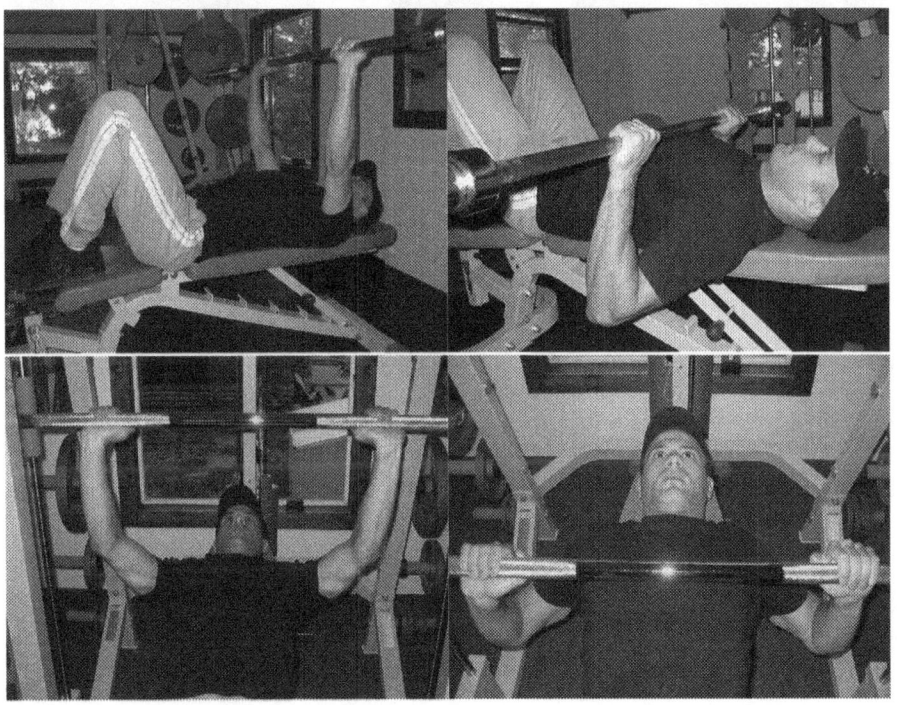

Dumbbell Presses
- more stabilizer muscles are required with this exercise
- trace an upside down "U" in the air

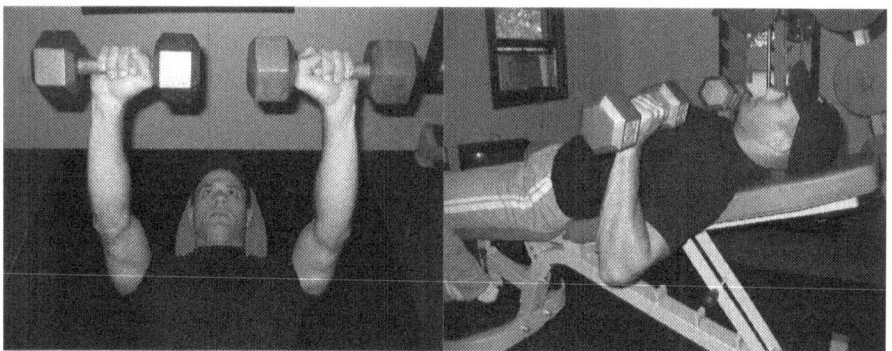

Dumbbell Fly
- same body position as dumbbell presses, just   - do not let hands drop below shoulders
  turn palms in
- simulate motion of hugging a large tree

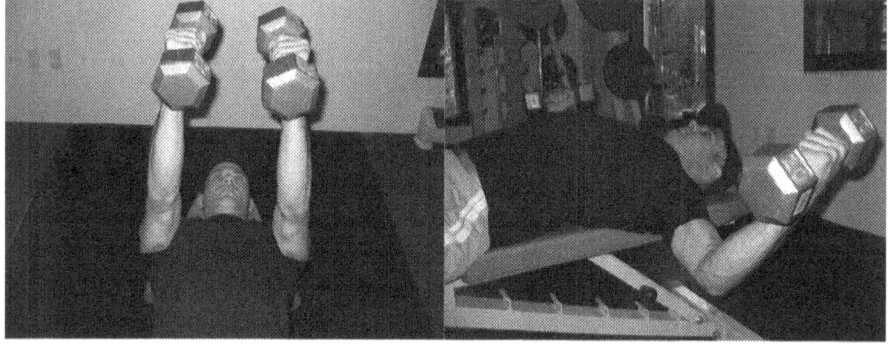

Push-ups
- keep your torso flat as a board
- do not drop your head
- advanced on toes

- lower yourself down, getting the chest close to the floor, then push back up
- modified on knees

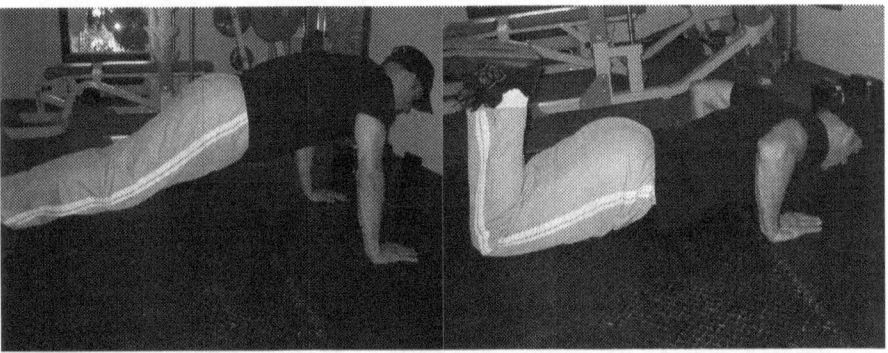

Lat Pull down
- lean back slightly, keep eyes up
- hand grip should be shoulder width or wider

- pull elbows diagonally down & backwards
- squeeze shoulder blades together
- pull bar down to top of chest

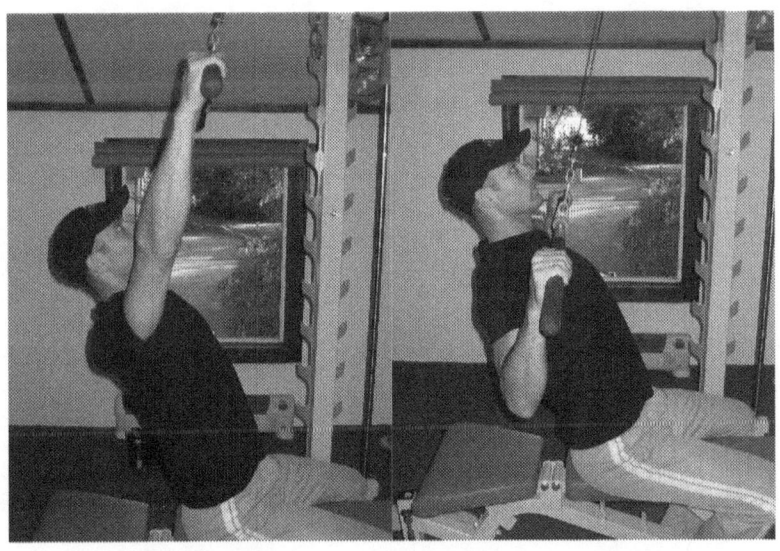

Seated Row
- sit up tall, only minimal torso movement is acceptable
- Pull elbows straight back, squeeze shoulder blades together

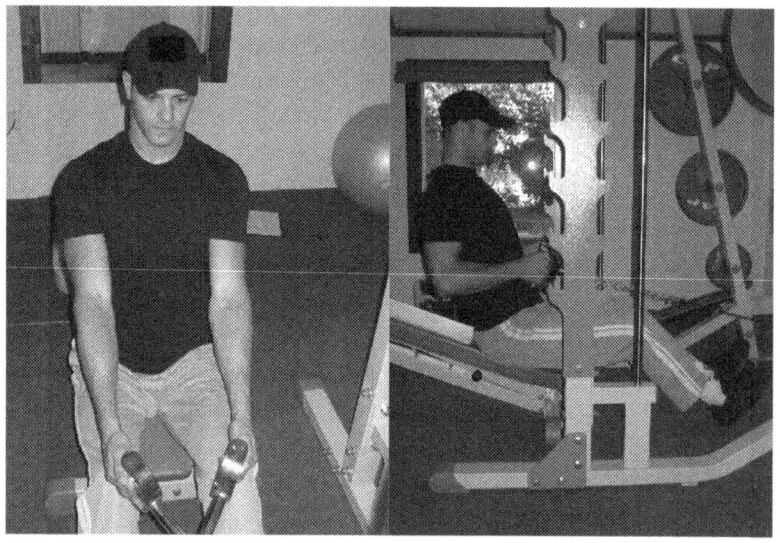

Reverse Fly
- use bench to support your lower back
- press hips and stomach into bench
- see Bent Over Rows for advanced body position
- swing arms out to the side, palms facing in
- squeeze shoulder blades together
- lift chest up slightly off bench

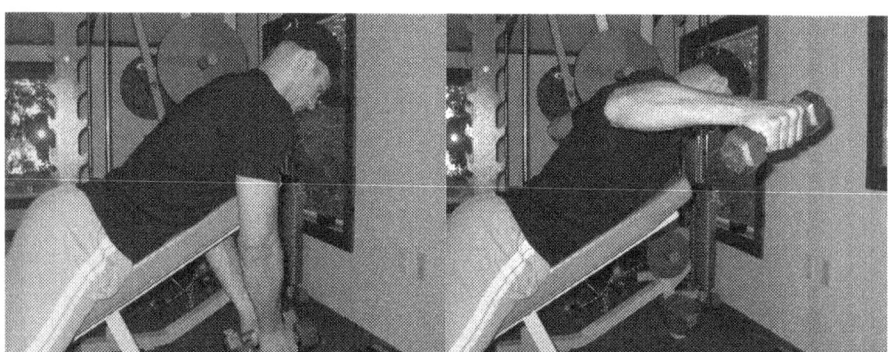

Bent Over Rows
- keep upper body at approximately 45° angle
- use lower back muscles to hold spine in neutral position
- can also be done with dumbbells
- sit back on heels, center of gravity should be hips and butt
- pull bar up to lower ribs, keep elbows out

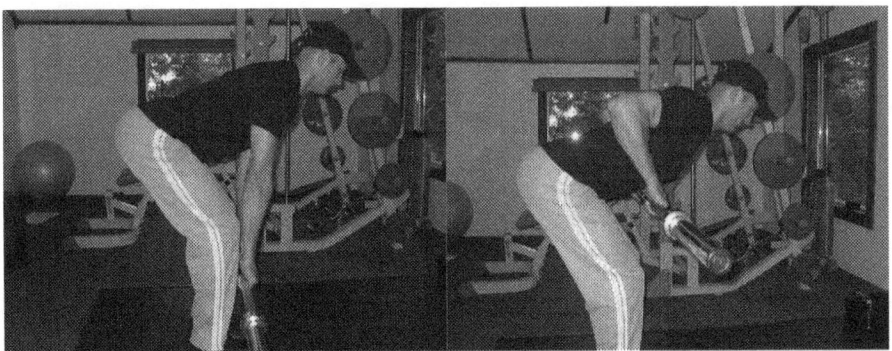

Note: If you experience any lower back pain with this exercise you can modify it by using dumbbells and lying on the bench in the same position as the Reverse Fly.

Squats (can be done with smith machine, barbell, dumbbells, or exercise ball)
- keep eyes up, head up, and shoulders back
- place bar on upper back (may want to use padding)
- place feet shoulder width apart
- sit hips back as you lower weight down
- keep knees behind the toes
- raise back up when thighs are parallel to floor

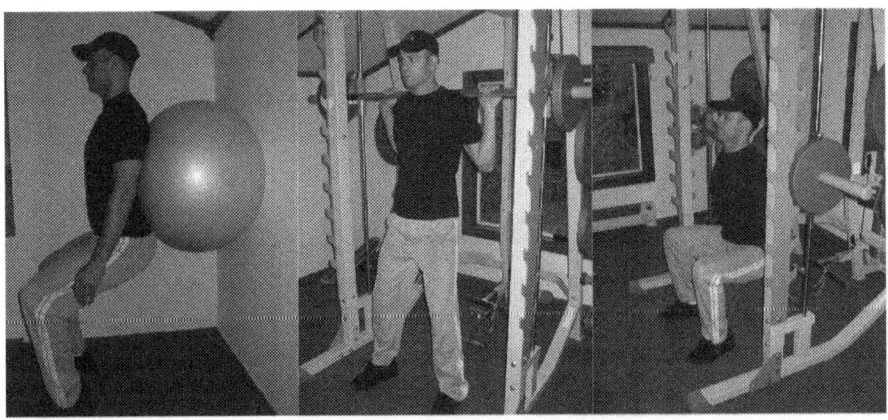

Lunges (can be done with smith machine, dumbbells, or no weights at all)
- choose from reverse (pictured), walking, or stationary
- keep most of your weight on heel of front leg
- lunges are not for beginners or those with knee injuries
- keep front knee behind toes
- lower self down until front thigh is parallel to floor

starting position   step back, weight on front leg   press back up using front leg

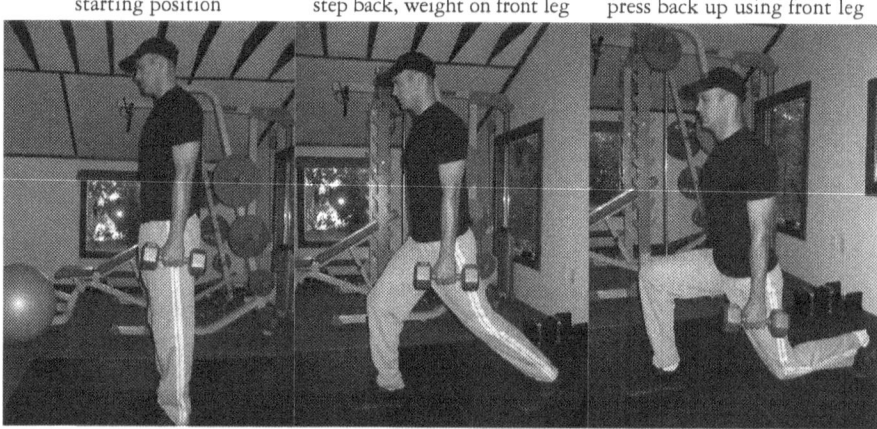

Note: It is highly recommended that you seek professional assistance in learning to perform this exercise correctly. Knee injuries can occur if performed improperly.

Ball Leg Curls
- place feet on top center of ball 4 inches apart
- keep body straight and use arms to stabilize
- roll ball while lifting hip upwards

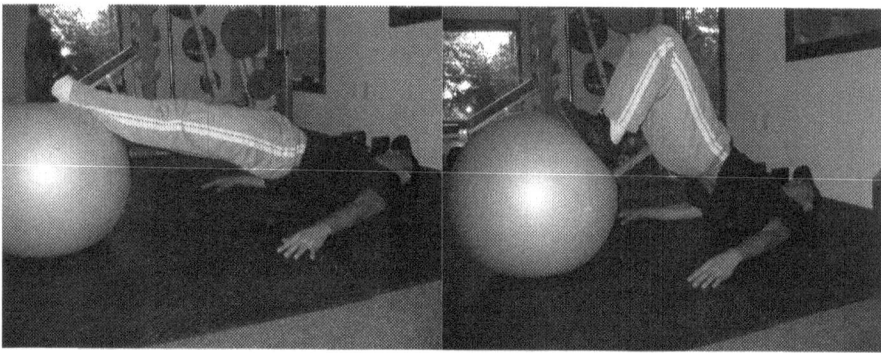

Calves (Heel Raises)
- you can use almost any stable object for these (steps are great)
- place feet so that your toes are up on the step, with the heels hanging off
- lower heels down as far as you can stretch, then raise up on your toes as high as possible

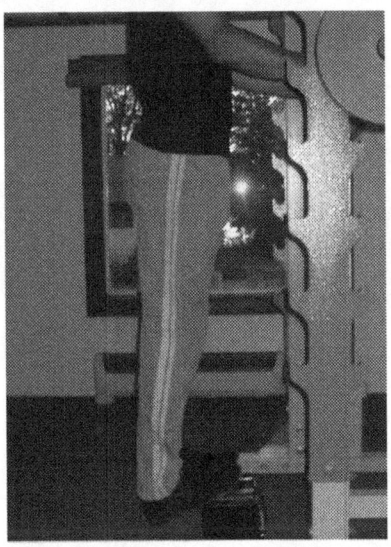

Shoulder Press (machine or dumbbells)
- start with hands at ear level, press up directly overhead
- keep shoulders against backrest
- trace the upside down "U" in the air
- can also be performed standing

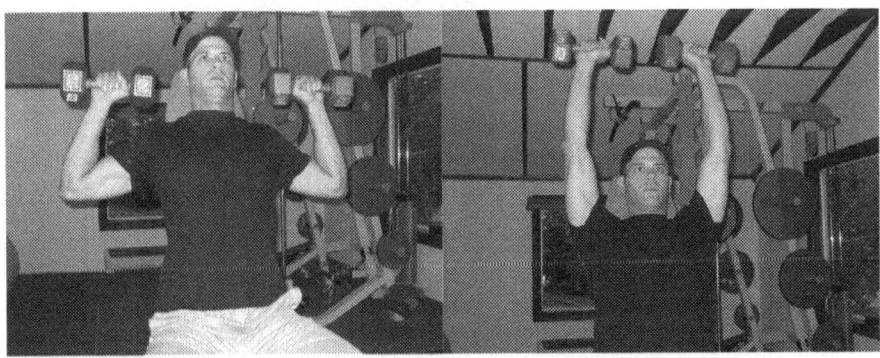

Lateral Raise
- raise hands to shoulder level and lower down to hips slowly, do not shrug shoulders

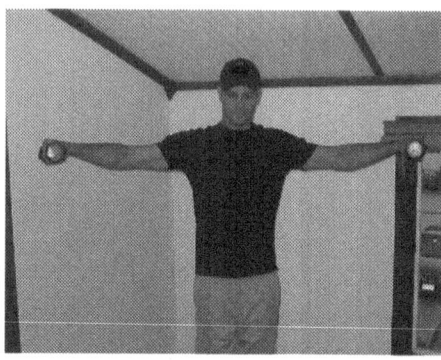

Triceps pushdowns
- keep elbows at sides, press down to full extension (squeeze muscle)
- raise hands back up to chest level, keeping elbows back

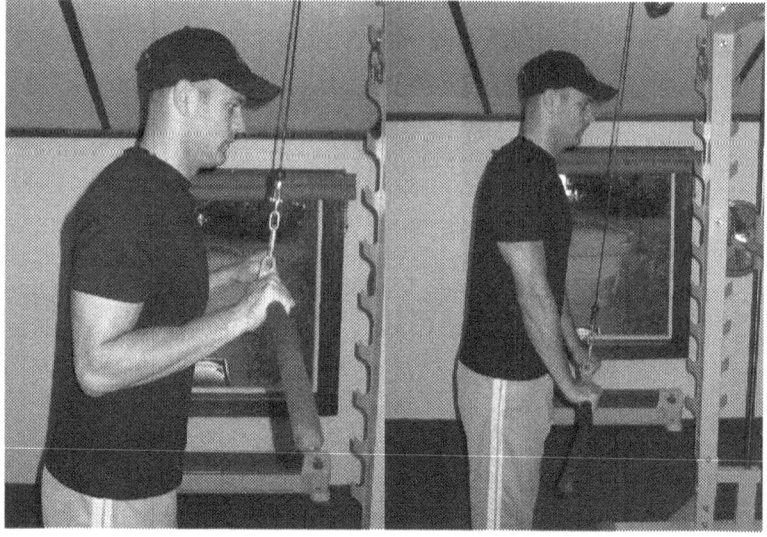

Skull crushers (cable machine or free weights)
- keep elbows pointing up and close together
- slowly lower weight towards your head
- raise back up, squeeze muscle at top, repeat

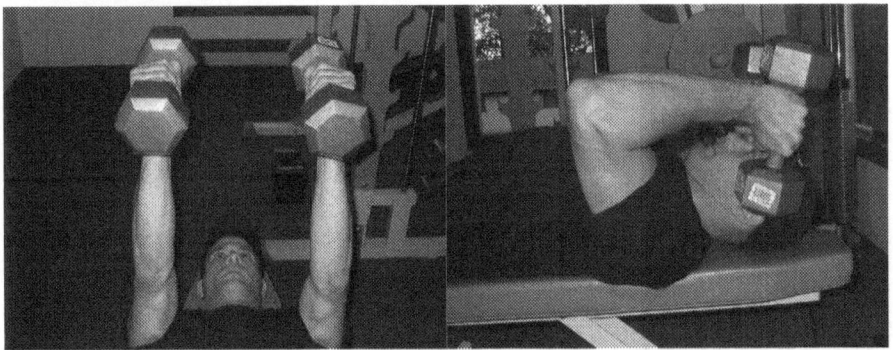

Kickbacks
- keep elbow high & against your side   - raise hand up & back, squeezing triceps at the
                                            top

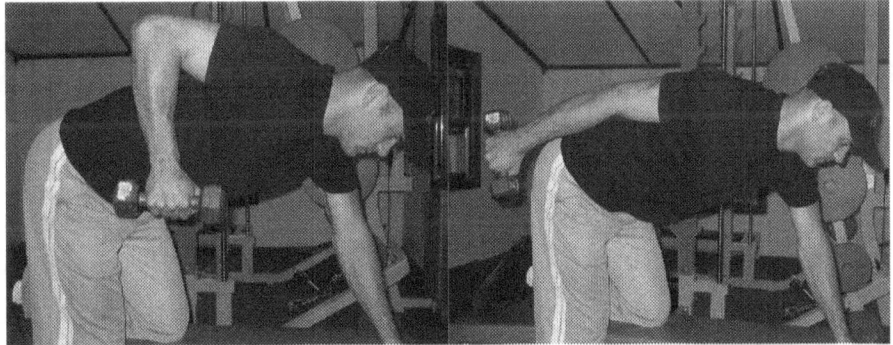

Dips
- focus on bending your elbows, not how low you can go
- keep body close to bench as you lower yourself down
- do not allow shoulders to drop below elbows
- press back up to start position

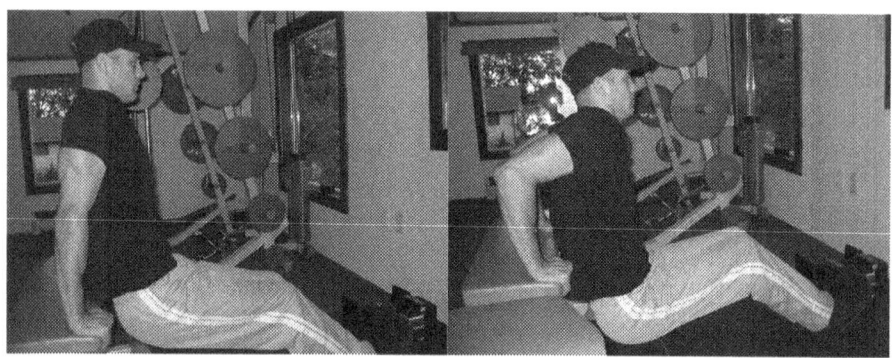

Biceps (hammer curl pictured below)
- keep elbows at sides and do not lift them forward
- do not allow arms to relax (fully extended)
- squeeze the biceps as much as you can at the top of each rep

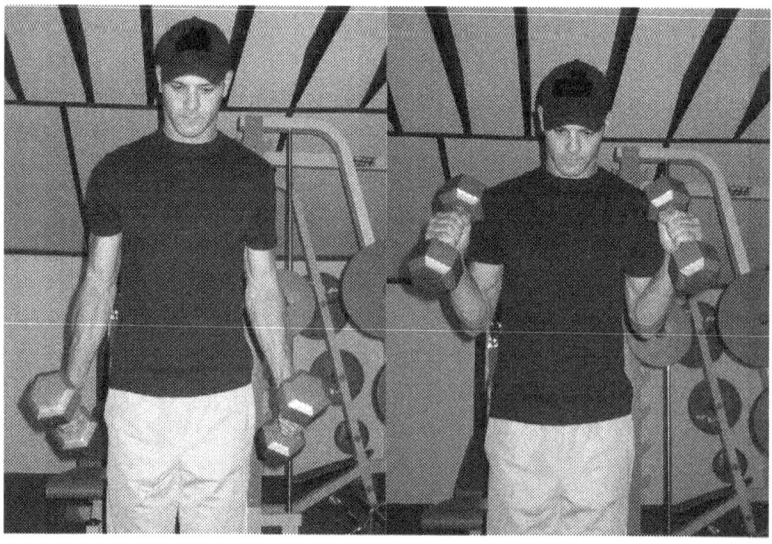

Abdominals (follow these basic rules for all)
- move slow and controlled, squeezing the muscles at the top of the motion
- quality not quantity, perform 2–3 sets of 2–3 different exercises (20–30 rep range each)
- do not hold your breath
- 3–4 days per week is plenty, you do not need to train abs everyday

basic crunch	modified basic crunch

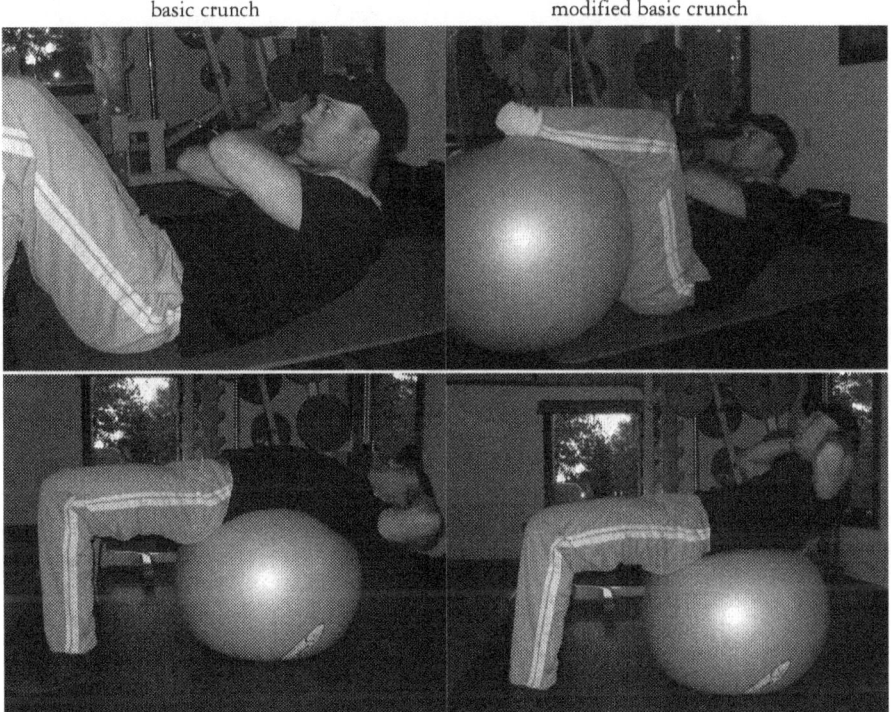

Ball crunch	keep hips elevated for best results

Stretching:

Maintaining and improving flexibility is something that most people need to do. This will allow your body to maintain its natural range of motion for performing activities as well as reduce chances of injury. There are three ideal times to stretch the body; all are when the body is warm.

1. During (in between sets) or after a weight workout. Target the muscles being worked.

2. After a cardio workout.

3. During or after a hot bath or shower.

The reason you want to stretch at these times is the muscles, ligaments, and tendons become more elastic when they are warm (like silly putty) and you will get greater range of motion out of them. The following is a list of stretches to cover the major muscle groups. All stretches should be held for 10–30 seconds and repeated at least once.

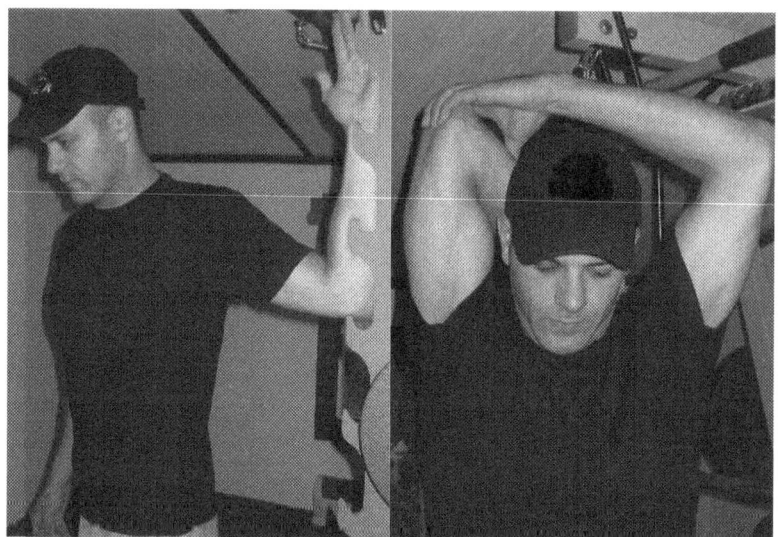

Chest—doorway stretch   Triceps—overhead stretch

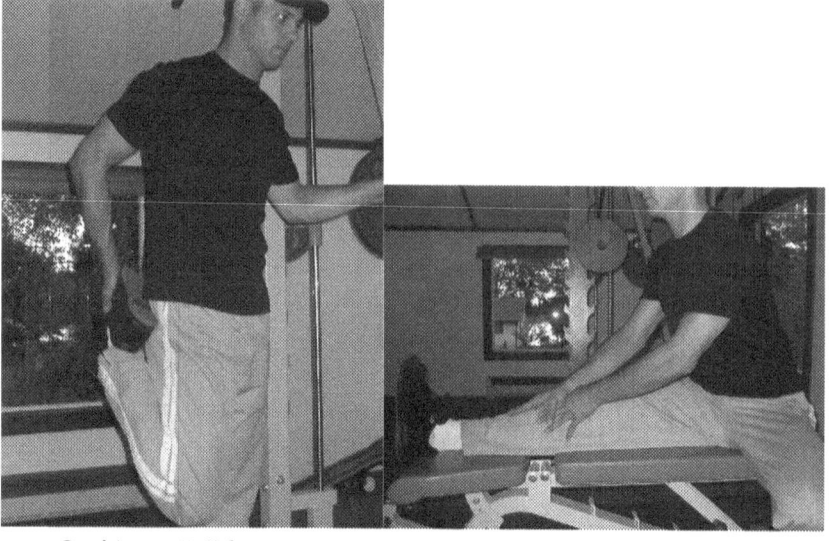

Quadriceps—Pull foot up   hamstrings—Reach for toes

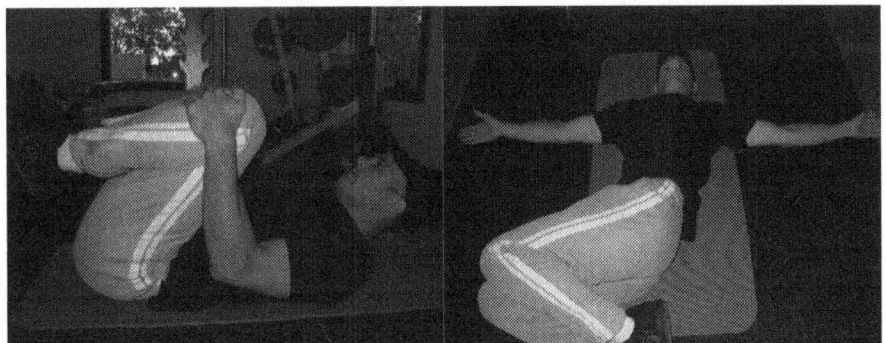

Lower back/trunk—knees to chest and drop knees side to side

Injuries and dangerous exercises:

As far as injuries are concerned, you can usually work around most of them without causing further damage. Sometimes you can even perform a particular exercise with a limited range of motion to prevent aggravation of an injury (new or old). Injuries can occur when one begins an exercise program. They generally happen in two ways. It is common for old injuries to resurface as you begin to place greater demands on your body. The injury was always there, you just did not recognize it because you have not used your body in this way for a long time. Avoid progressing your workouts too fast and you can minimize this type of injury. The second way injuries can occur is from poor technique or dangerous exercises. If you do not feel you completely understand the pictures and descriptions of the above listed exercises, it will be well worth the money to hire someone to ensure you do them properly. As far as dangerous exercises are concerned, protecting the shoulder is a high priority. The shoulder complex is a ball and socket joint allowing for a greater range of motion than most others. This makes it a less stable joint and prone to injury if not conditioned properly. An injury to the shoulder can affect many daily activities, here are a few exercises you should avoid to reduce the risk.

1. Lat Pull downs behind the neck. Many people perform these safely for years without ever having a problem. Proponents claim this exercise targets the back better than the front pull down. After reviewing the risks to the shoulder complex, the risks do not outweigh the benefits.

2. Upright Rows, this is an exercise you commonly see for targeting the trapezius and deltoid muscles. It also puts the shoulder complex at risk. A shoulder shrug and side/lateral raise will safely target these muscle groups.

3. Shoulder/Military Press (behind the head), another one that places undue stress on the shoulder complex. This exercise should be performed to the front of the head or with dumbbells.

Appendix VI

Health Logs

I have included an example of the logs I use for tracking aerobic workouts and weight training workouts for my clients. I highly recommend you use these to monitor your progress. You should also record your food intake. You can use any journal and simply write down the foods you are eating. It works even better if you actually plan the meals out in advance. I like my clients to use a number system for their hunger level. I use a scale of 1–3, 1 meaning you were not very hungry going into that meal and 3 meaning you were extremely hungry before that meal. If you have 3's at certain times of the day you may need to increase the size of the previous meal or decrease the time between meals to fix this. You do not want to be extremely hungry before each meal because this can lead to overeating. Always review your journal to find where you need to make improvements to your diet.

The cardio log is something you simply fill in and look at after a few weeks and be able to tell right away if you have been doing everything you can and should to reach your goal. Use this log to monitor your workouts and keep track of your frequency, intensity, and duration. Progress your routine when it is time

The weight training log is also very important, this will help you to remember all the different weights you are using for each exercise as well as let you know when it is time to increase the resistance. If you notice you are hitting the high end of your rep range for all three sets, it may be time to increase the weights. However, make sure you can do the exercise with proper form before increasing any weights. The sample days provided should give you an understanding of how to record your workouts.

CARDIO TRACKING LOG

Wk 1	Type	Time	HR	Wk 2	Type	Time	HR
M				M			
T				T			
W				W			
Th				Th			
F				F			
Sat				Sat			
Sun				Sun			
Wk 3	Type	Time	HR	Wk 4	Type	Time	HR
M				M			
T				T			
W				W			
Th				Th			
F				F			
Sat				Sat			
Sun				Sun			

Weight Training Log

Exercise					Workout # 2			Workout # 3			Workout # 4		
		1	2	3	1	2	3	1	2	3	1	2	3
Phase Ia													
Chest Press	WT	20	20	20	20	20	20	20	25	20			
	Reps	18	16	15	20	19	17	20	17	17			
Leg Extension	WT	25	25	25	30	30	30	30	35	30			
	Reps	20	20	20	20	18	17	20	15	16			
Lat Pulldown	WT	30	30	30	30	35	30	35	35	30			
	Reps	20	18	17	20	15	16	18	15	16			
Ball squat	WT	0	0	0	0	0	0	5	5	0			
	Reps	18	16	14	20	17	14	20	15	15			
Lateral Raise	WT	3	3	3	3	3	3	3	3	3			
	Reps	16	13	12	18	16	15	20	16	15			
Tricep Pushdown	WT	20	20	20	20	25	25	25	25	25			
	Reps	20	18	17	20	17	15	17	15	14			
Dumbbell Curl	WT	8	8	8	8	8	8	8	10	8			
	Reps	19	17	14	20	18	15	20	14	15			
Lowback bridges	WT												
	Reps	6	5	4	8	6	5	10	8	6			
Sample Week		M	T	W	T	F	S	S					
	*	W	off	C	C	W	C	C					
* W = weights C = cardio													

Weight Training Log Workout # 2 Workout # 3 Workout # 4

Phase II		1	2	3	1	2	3	1	2	3	1	2	3
Workout A													
Incline Press	WT	25			25	30	30	30	30	25			
	Reps	15	14	13	17	15	12	16	14	12			
Dumbbell Fly	WT	10			10			10	12	10			
	Reps	14	13	13	16	13	13	17	14	14			
Overhead Press	WT	10			10			10					
	Reps	15	12	10	16	13	12	17	15	14			
Lateral Raise	WT	5			5			5					
	Reps	15	14	12	18	14	12	18	15	13			
Rope Pulldowns	WT	25			25			25		30			
	Reps	13	12	10	15	14	12	17	15	9			
Ab Crunches	WT												
	Reps	20	18	17	20	17	15	17	15	14			
Sample Week		M	T	W	T	F	S	S					
	*	A	C	B	C	off	A/C	C					

* A = workout A, B = workout B, C = cardio workout

Appendix VII

Vitamins, minerals, and supplements

Overview: Several large studies have been conducted and reviewed by various experts in the field of cardiology. They concluded there is no evidence that vitamin supplementation reduces the risk of cardiovascular disease. *Health, October, 2003 p 54.* They reviewed studies using the supplementation of vitamins A, C, E, beta-carotene; and antioxidant or multivitamin combinations. More research is being conducted to confirm these findings, until then you can use them as an added insurance plan, but do not rely on them. The doctors who reviewed the studies were shocked at these findings as you also may be. The conclusion, we need to come, is that we all must increase our intake of fruits and vegetables to get these nutrients in their natural form along with all the enzymes and fiber. Vitamin and mineral supplements can be used as added insurance, but not as our primary source for these nutrients. As for supplements used for increased sports performance (ergogenic aids), aside from a few exceptions, you are better off without these expensive products.

Calcium: (National Osteoporosis Foundation) recommends women age 19–50, 1000 milligrams/day (1500 for osteoporosis prevention). You may have already learned from the news, or various product commercials that the latest research also shows calcium can help with fat loss. While this may be true, there are a few things you should know about it. Your body cannot absorb calcium in high doses. You should therefore meet your intake requirement through several small doses throughout the day limiting them to no more than 500 milligrams per dose. There are various types of calcium supplements out there, although foods such as dairy products and dark green leafy vegetables (spinach and broccoli) are probably your best source due to a better absorption factor. For example, a 600 milligram supplement only contains 240 milligrams of elemental calcium which is about the same as 1 cup of milk. Supplements should be used to help you fill in the gaps and reach your daily requirement. There are several types of calcium supplements including calcium carbonate, calcium citrate, calcium phosphate, and coral calcium. The latest research is proving coral calcium to be nothing but hype. Do not waste your money on this significantly more expensive version which offers no advantage over the others.

Sodium: The current RDA listed on your food labels set the level at 2,400 milligrams per day. The latest research shows that we take in more than this level despite the fact that we should really reduce intake to 1,500 milligrams per day. Most Americans take in too much sodium and not enough potassium. This imbalance can increase blood pressure which leads to many other health problems. Food makers are fighting against these new guidelines because they care more about you liking the food than your health. You can easily hit near 5000 mg per day just from eating "normal foods" during the day and having a single frozen meal (1,000 mg) and one can of condensed soup (2,500 mg) for dinner. For more information on this see *Lauran Neergaard's AP article "Report Urges Americans to Reduce Sodium" 2/12/04.*

Creatine: One of the few proven supplements that can increase (specific) performance in an exercising individual. There have been numerous studies on this supplement for many years. They have tested it for a wide range of purposes. Here is what we know: It will improve performance in short-burst, anaerobic exercises (weight lifting, sprinting). It helps the individual to increase body mass by increasing lean muscle and water weight (water attaches to new muscle). While this may be desirable or advantageous for some individuals, it is not for all. This increased body weight can actually be a handicap for endurance type athletes. There are a number of studies in recent years showing that it may produce benefits in many other aspects of our health, but until more research comes out, I will not comment any further on them. One thing you should also know about is the question regarding the safety of using creatine. There is some evidence that there are potential kidney problems related to creatine use. Some individuals also experience abdominal cramping and bloating. These side effects and potential dangers were enough for some sports programs to discontinue its use. Use creatine at your own risk.

Androstenedione & Androstenediol: The latest research shows that strength trainers given a dose of this supposed testosterone enhancer showed no signs of increased testosterone. However, they did find significant increased levels of estrogen. This would produce the opposite effect of what most taking this supplement would want.

Ephedra: (Ma Huang/related stimulants) When clients ask about these products, I ask them if they enjoy the feeling of their heart beating out of their chest. Ephedra and related stimulants basically do one thing; they artificially elevate your heart rate and your metabolism (temporarily) and allow your body to burn a few extra calories. They may also allow you to workout harder as well. Enough people have had heart complications while doing this that it was finally pulled off the market. These types of products as well as all the carb and fat blockers are used as crutches because people are afraid to rely on their own ability to stick to a plan. Avoid these products, get your act together and you'll do just fine.

Nutrient (Fat or Carb) Blockers: They come in various forms, all claiming you can eat whatever you want and just take a dose of their product and you won't have to worry about the excess calorie or fat ingestion. First of all, there is virtually no proof (independently controlled studies) that these products work (have a significant effect). However, they do have some possible side effects. Many times these products contain the word "chito" which comes from chitin, which they are made with. Chitin comes from shellfish. If you have any allergies to shellfish this could present a problem. Another problem is that they can reduce your body's absorption of fat soluble vitamins (A, D, E, & K). Long term use could lead to health problems.

Caffeine: While this is also a stimulant, it is (depending on dosage) a milder one which many are addicted to and taking anyway. There are scientific studies that show caffeine can both help burn fat, and aid in delaying fatigue during exercise. While these effects are significant, they are not all that remarkable and they only come with small doses. Drinking coffee is also not a good thing because it contains certain ingredients that can increase cortisol secretions and promote fat storage. Green tea would be a healthier choice.

Chromium picolinate: Once believed to help with fat loss and muscle gain, this supplement has been extensively studied. The latest research shows that this popular supplement does not work.

Protein: This is probably the most commonly used supplement despite the fact that most people can meet all of their needs through natural foods alone. So why do so many people use protein supplements if they can get it from natural sources? Time and appetite. It can be much more convenient to make a shake or eat a bar versus cooking up a chicken breast. Another advantage of protein supplements is you typically do not get as much fat per serving. Those who are getting protein through natural foods must make sure they use lean sources to avoid taking in too much fat. If you remember the milk example in chapter 4, 1% milk has the same amount of protein as 2%, it just has less fat. Protein supplements can also make it easier to control the types of protein sources you take in (whey, soy, casein, milk, egg). Whey protein is a great choice for a post workout smoothie because it gets digested more rapidly. Casein protein releases into the blood stream more slowly and would make a good evening protein source. There are different benefits from each protein source which go beyond the scope of this book. The best thing you can do is to make sure you eat a variety of foods and you will then get multiple types of nutrients from them.

References

Essentials of Strength Training and Conditioning (NSCA), edited by Thomas R. Baechle, 1994

Nutrition for Fitness and Sport, Melvin H. Williams, 1995

Quantitative Analysis of Single- vs. Multiple- set Programs in Resistance Training (Journal of Strength and Conditioning Research) Feb 2004 p 35

The New Encyclopedia of Modern Bodybuilding: The Bible of Bodybuilding, Arnold Scharzenegger with Bill Dobbins, 1999

The NO-Grain Diet, Dr. Joseph Mercola, 2003

978-0-595-37659-9
0-595-37659-2